Cancer Babble

by

Chris Drnaso

Cover Illustration:
© Can Stock Photo / Kubko
csp47384290
Large JPEG (3000x2399 px - 300 dpi)
©Kubko - Can Stock Photo Inc.
June 9, 2020
Order Id : 5998787
<!-- HTML Credit Code for Can Stock Photo -->
<a href="https://www.canstockphoto.com">(c) Can Stock Photo / Kubko</a>

Author's Photo: Ean Adams

ISBN: 9798652248765
Imprint: Independently published
Library of Congress Control Number: 2020910652
Published by: Chris Drnaso
Palos Hills, IL.

To

Marilyn

My Wife,
My Best Friend,
My Caregiver

Also by Chris Drnaso

CLEARING

THORN

MANAGING HENRY

A PRAIRIE FORTNIGHT

Introduction

I'm not sure where to start for a couple of reasons. One, I never wrote a book about me before, and secondly, my cancer story started quite a while ago. So I guess I'll begin with the first one; writing about myself. There's a credo that many writers subscribe to; *'write about what you know'* and as it turns out, I know about me, and as you'll come to find out in these pages, I know about cancer.

I wrote most of this introduction months ago, but today I am circling back to look at it from a fresh perspective. You might be surprised at how few writers work from an outline and that would describe my own process. When I sit down to write a book, I have only the sketchiest idea of where the story might be headed. I don't worry about it as I have come to believe that, *'the keyboard knows what to do'*.

If I'm going to write about me, maybe I should tell you a little about me. I was born in 1953 in a neighborhood called Clearing on the southwest side of Chicago. Never heard of it? I thought not. Maybe this will help; if you can find Midway Airport, you can find Clearing. I married my college sweetheart and best friend Marilyn in 1982. I had two parents, two sisters, and two sons. I've been a Chicagoan my entire life. Not only that, I've always lived in the same general area on the southwest side and have only had five addresses since birth. I was the 'cable-guy' for thirty five years before retiring at the end of 2016 shortly before my 64th birthday. I started writing at age sixty and have published four novels over the past six years. There's one other thing you should know; I get cancer a lot. Three times; that seems like a lot to me anyway.

Well, that was succinct. I guess you can see now why I never wrote about me before...I just told you my life history in 145 words. In truth, I could have scaled it down to under a hundred words without breaking a sweat.

There are two things I know about; writing and getting cancer. I guess that's a good thing as this is a book about life with cancer.

Indulge me while I talk about writing for a moment. I mentioned during my brief biography above that I have written four novels over the past six years. The first, *CLEARING*, is about four teens coming of age during the 1960s in the southwest side Chicago neighborhood of Clearing. It is true that

I grew up in Clearing in the 1960s, but as I have explained numerous times, *CLEARING* is not autobiographical. My biography above was less than 150 words and *CLEARING* weighed in at 116,000 words. Do the math. *CLEARING* was all about; *Write about what you know*, right? I'm going to stick to that same doctrine during *CANCER BABBLE*. Whereas *CLEARING* was never about me, *CANCER BABBLE* has a lot to do with me.

Do you want to hear more about my writing? I didn't think so. If you are inclined, I have an author's page on Amazon with links to more information. This book isn't about those books, so let's move on.

So, if a book called *CANCER BABBLE* caught your attention, my guess is that it means one of a couple of things.

- You have or had cancer
- You know or knew someone with cancer
- Your Zodiac sign is Cancer, and you are a complete idiot.

The first two bullet points above, sadly, apply to close to 100% of the people on Earth. It's damn near impossible to find anyone anywhere who hasn't had cancer impact their life. That's a sobering thought, and even though I have no data to back up that claim, I'll leave it stand as my sense is that it is the truth.

Say what you want about cancer, it doesn't discriminate. Cancer doesn't care if you are short, tall, thin, fat, smart, or dumb. Cancer doesn't care about your race or your religion; it doesn't care if you are a nice person or a complete asshole. Men, women, and children; no one is immune.

Sometimes, it helps me to think of cancer as a person as compared to a thing. These personifications aren't meant to humanize the beast, but to me, they make cancer more beatable; more controllable. I may hate cancer, but it seems that cancer is very fond of me. If cancer was a person, and that person had a nice home in the suburbs, and within this nice home there was a family room, and in this family room there was a fireplace, and above this fireplace there was a mantle; cancer would have a framed picture of me placed prominently upon this mantle. Whenever his cancer buddies would come over, invariably someone would look at my picture, and ask, "Who's this putz?"

Cancer would get all excited and say, "That guy? He's one of my favorites." And then he'd go on and tell them how he'd been jerking me around for the past fourteen years.

I was diagnosed with my first cancer in 2006, and yesterday, June 10th, 2019, I started treatment in my third battle with cancer.

Before you say, "Oh crap, this guy's writing another *'poor me, I got cancer'*, book," I promise you that if you catch me in any moments of self-pity or self-wallowing you have my permission to toilet paper the trees in front of my house. There are many people out there that want or need your sympathy, but I'm not one of them. I've had a full and wonderful life for a guy with a paltry 145 word biography. I've made my peace with that.

I will however talk honestly and openly with you about life with cancer. Talk is the key word in this sentence. All books adopt a certain voice; a narrator's voice. I have reread this book several times and realize that *CANCER BABBLE* has adopted an unusual voice. It reads like a conversation; so much so that I almost added the subtitle *CANCER BABBLE; A Conversation*, but in the end, I did not.

I have worked hard to find the funny in cancer. It would be tragedy to go through cancer three times over fourteen years and not find the humor in it.

As a warning, there are moments that any story with cancer at its core can turn dark. I hope at those moments, it doesn't sound like I'm complaining or whining. Keep in mind, I'm a guy who has heard the words, *"You've got cancer"* three times, and I'm still vertical. That being the case, I don't think I've got the right to bitch about anything.

Cancer Babble

Table of Contents

Interlude One: He's wrong.

So what the hell is an Interlude? Good question. Most of my story follows a chronological beginning to end pattern starting in 2006. An Interlude tells you what's happening in the present. Why would I do something like that? I don't know, but the truth is I couldn't figure out a better way to flip from the past to the present. I hope, Dear Reader, that you are OK with that.

Spring, 2019. I'm not sure of the exact date and, in truth, it's probably not important. It's funny in life how some things can be not a big deal, and then, in the blink of an eye, they become a big deal. In the spring of 2019, there appears to be a small amount of blood in my urine. This is so not a big deal, but blood in the urine is still blood in the urine and most medical professionals, as well as a none-to-bright lay person like me, would agree that blood should not be in one's urine. Having had my prostate removed due to cancer in July of 2018, (a scant eight months ago), I am convinced that this is just another of the myriad side effects that I've had to deal with since that traitorous and pesky prostate gland was removed. Good riddance, I say.

Believing I have nothing more than a urinary tract infection (UTI), I contact my urologist's office and ask if they would be kind enough to write an order for a urinalysis. This should be easy. I'll go for the urinalysis, followed by a healthy dose of antibiotics, the blood goes away, and I get on with my life. What, may I ask you, could be simpler?

That thing I said earlier, about how in life some things can be not a big deal and then they become a big deal, is about to come full circle. Instead of an order for a urinalysis, I received a call from my urologist. He immediately starts throwing around the 'C' word. I'm not ready to hear that word again for a long time; preferably never. I'm still dealing with issues from my last bout with cancer. Simply stated, he's wrong. There is no way this is cancer. I believe in my heart that he's wrong about this. I hope he's wrong; I pray he's wrong.

Chapter One-Support

Because I'm not sure where to start this discussion, let's talk about support first. Support seems like a safe place to wade into these cancerous waters. You've been told you have cancer, and suddenly, all those things that seemed so important to you yesterday don't seem too important anymore. You're scared, you're angry, you're upset, but you are not alone.

The American Cancer Society hosts hundreds of Relay for Life events every summer, and I strongly suggest that if you are a cancer survivor, or caregiver, or a supporter that you attend a Relay. I've made it a point to attend at least one of these events each year since 2007. Survivors are given a purple tee shirt. Go to a Relay and look at some of the people in purple tees. There is nothing as heartbreaking as seeing children, some in strollers, wearing purple. It is a powerful message about who is blessed and who has drawn a really bad hand. Relay for Life events are special for another reason, they are meant as a celebration. It's even part of the Relay's catchphrase; *Celebrate, Remember, Fight Back.* Cancer all too often has more than its share of gloom and doom attached to it. Relays put a different spin on it. Go on-line, find a Relay near you, and experience it for yourself. God bless the American Cancer Society (ACS). The ACS is one of many organizations that offer support for those dealing with cancer.

Beyond ACS, there are lots of cancer support groups. Churches and hospitals oftentimes will sponsor groups. There are even specific groups you can join where you can interact with people dealing with the same type of cancer that you have.

I chose the latter, and in 2007, after my diagnosis of anal cancer, I joined a support group with others whose anus had also betrayed them. Anal cancer is considered to be the 'clown prince' of cancers...arguably the funniest of all cancers. For those who flunked biology, that's the one where your butt hurts.

People don't like to think of it this way, but there's a pecking order to cancer and anal cancer is not high on the pecking order list. We discussed this in our support group, and we decided we were going to change that culture. We began planning a walk-a-thon. What better way to raise awareness? After all, hardly any causes have walk-a-thons, right?

If by some chance any of the 12 people who showed up for our walk-a-thon should read this book, I would like to say, 'thank you for your support'. It didn't go well ...hardly anyone showed up...we raised a total of $81.00 which didn't even come close to covering the bar bill after the walk.

It wasn't for lack of effort; we really did try our best.

Take this for example. There are causes that adopt a certain color to help people identify with their cause. Pink is by far the most iconic example. If you see pink, you think of breast cancer, (or if you're a moron, Owens-Corning Fiberglass Insulation). We figured we would try that, so we decided on a color and had tee-shirts made up. I'm not going to tell you what color we picked for our cause. All I'm going to say is, *"What were we thinking?"*

Our ideas seemed to go from bad to worse. Someone suggested that a slogan might help people identify with our cause. Years later, as I look back it's hard to believe we actually considered some of these suggestions for a slogan:

- "Anal Cancer: Get Behind a Great Cause"
- "Anal Cancer: We'll Crack This Yet!"

Several suggestions bordered on being Zen-like:

- "The Hole is Greater than the Sum of its Parts"
- "There is a Light at the end of the Darkest Tunnel"

But finally, after much debate, the back of our tee shirts read:

- "Rectum?...It Damn Near Killed Him"

It wasn't all bad. In fact we had offers from two companies who were interested in being our corporate sponsor. We politely declined the offer from the Roto-Rooter people, but I did want to thank the people at Charmin for their sponsorship. Charmin was very generous. They made up goody-bags for all the walkers and included some of their most popular and absorbent products.

In retrospect, one of the worst things about anal cancer was living in fear of alien abduction. There seems to be a lot of rectal probing in an alien abduction. No thank you, I was already getting plenty of that.

OK, it's time for full disclosure. I tend to make stuff up, but keep in mind that I'm a writer; a storyteller; a fabricator. On that note, none of that stuff I wrote about the walk-a-thon to raise awareness for anal cancer is true.

The real truth is, in 2007, going through cancer for the first time, I was scared. Cancer is scary, but it was less scary on the days that I had the ability to laugh at cancer. I tried to look at cancer like it was the bully in the schoolyard. If you can laugh at the bully, it empowers you. Cancer is not a sacred cow, and if it's OK with you, I'd like to spend as much time in this book as I can thumbing my nose at cancer. I want to put a thumb tack on cancer's chair. I'd like you to join me when I go to cancer's house and leave a bag of flaming poop on his doorstep.

Now, on the other end of the cancer pecking order spectrum is breast cancer. I was awed the first time I attended a breast cancer fundraiser with my wife. I went expecting to see wailing and gnashing of teeth but there was none of that. As horrible as cancer is, and I can only imagine how devastating it is for a woman to go through breast cancer, these brave women put aside their angst and their grief and celebrated life. Many group members carried pictures of a mother or aunt or sister or friend who had fought and lost the battle, but I saw no look of despair on the faces of the women carrying these pictures. Instead, there was a look of steely resolve and determination in their eyes. Every man, woman, and child had a reason to be at that event, and I'm sure many of those reasons were tragic, but for those few hours the collective thought was, SCREW YOU CANCER.

Laughter outweighed tears as humor was a huge part of the event. Tee shirts and signage that read 'Save Second Base' and 'Save the Ta-Tas' were everywhere along with numerous clever and inspirational messages. My favorite was a tee shirt that read, *'Of course they're fake...the real ones tried to kill me'*. Bras, mostly dyed pink, were everywhere. It was as if the participants challenged themselves to see how many uses they could come up with for their old bras. At several places along the walk, bras were strung across the street between trees. The fire hydrants wore bras, and in some cases skirts and tiaras. Bras were hung from flagpoles.

There was even one man walking around wearing a bra, but as it turned out he wasn't part of the event. He apparently was dealing with some separate issues. They asked him to leave.

And I think we all know why breast cancer gets so much support. Because they're BREASTS! "Breasts," (you can't see me now, but I have a dreamy faraway look of wonder and awe on my face as I whisper the word aloud). Breasts have always been an iconic part of the American landscape. I grew up in the mammary infatuated 1950s: *The Golden Age of Bosoms*. Thinking back on my youth, it was unfair for a young boy to be figuratively smacked in the face by a giant boob at every turn. Jane Mansfield and Marilyn Monroe were at the top of the Double-D list. Breasts are so mesmerizing that even Sophia Loren couldn't help but stare at Jayne Mansfield's impressive cleavage in a famous and iconic photograph from the era. Don't play dumb with me, you know damn well which picture I'm talking about.

Lest I linger too long on this subject let me bid adieu by asking, "Do you know who has a nice rack?" My Uncle Nuncio, I'm serious; if you can picture Sasquatch with about a 'B' cup that would give you a pretty good idea of what my uncle looks like. Nuncio, a sweet but clueless man, had no problem going outside and doing his yard work without a shirt on. I can picture him now. He's waving to the neighbors as he jiggles along on his riding lawn mower. It is a disturbing image to say the least. And the grief he caused my aunt; I can still hear her, "Nuncio...put a shirt on...there's enough suffering in the world."

I love my Uncle Nuncio, hairy boobs and all. Last year for his birthday I bought him a tee shirt...it read, *'Save the Ta-Tas'*.

Here we go again, I didn't have an Uncle Nuncio, but most of what I wrote about this breast cancer walk is true. It was therapeutic to see all these people who had been victimized by this disease gather together for a few hours to show their support for one another. Whether you have cancer or are caregiving for someone who does, remember this; there is support for you out there, and support is a big deal when going through cancer. No matter how powerful your resolve is on the first day of cancer you may find that this disease, in time, will wear down your tenacity.

You don't have to go through it alone.

The thought of anyone going through it alone is just plain sad.

Chapter Two-Doctor, Heal Thyself

Three little words...most cancer patients will tell you the worst thing you'll ever hear are those three little words, "You have cancer". That wasn't the case for me... the three little words that really got me down were Health Maintenance Organization, or as it is more commonly known, HMO. Do you know how this little insanity play works? No, well then it's a good thing I'm writing this book. In an HMO, your doctor becomes your 'Primary Care Physician' or PCP and his role is to 'refer' you to 'specialists' in the 'network'. The optimum word there is network. Remember this...in-network=good ...out-of-network=BAD.

I don't want to scare anyone, but I knew a guy who went out of the network and three days later they found his fat, bloated, pasty white body tossed into a dumpster. It had nothing to do with him going out of the network. He had a gambling problem and got crosswise with some bad people. My point is, he looked horrible and really should have taken better care of himself. Oh yeah, and one more thing, don't stray outside the network.

So I go see my PCP for a referral to an oncologist and I'm fortunate as sometimes your choices within the network can be very limited. I was lucky to have two to choose from, and even better, one was local...the other guy was in Beijing, China. I guess I should have been concerned when I went to see him for the first time and my GPS told me to *'take a right after turning into the trailer park'*. So anyway, I felt better when I got to his office; it was a very nice double-wide. Even better, I got the good parking space under the aluminum awning. It eased my angst when I saw that he had his diplomas on display. One wasn't actually a diploma...for some reason he had framed his membership into the *"Jelly of the Month Club"*. The other document was a college degree; he went to culinary school. That was OK; it still showed effort on his part. He wasn't a good doctor, but I kept going back because he was in the network and was such a wonderful baker. There comes a time in a relationship when you know it's time to part ways...that day for me was when I ran into him at Shop & Save and he was wearing a Jiffy Lube shirt.

Sorry, I'm making stuff up again. Most of the above is a fabrication except for this, the first time I went through cancer, I was in an HMO. That would have probably been OK except that my Primary Care Physician (PCP) was an incompetent moron. You will come to find out that I do a lot of name calling in this book. Childish? You bet. Maybe I should get tested for Tourette's syndrome?

I have had hemorrhoids since high school but, except for an occasional bad day, they were manageable. That was the case until 2005 when my rectal pain started to become an issue. I went to my PCP who told me it was a hemorrhoid and to just deal with it. He warned me that I would be making a big mistake if I was to pursue any type of treatment. I was in HMO hell. I needed a PCP referral to see someone else, and he was disinclined to send me to a specialist. So, on many days, I suffered in silence. Finally, after repeated visits where I groveled and begged for him to send me to a specialist, he acquiesced. In retrospect, I might have been wise to assume that an incompetent doctor would refer me to an incompetent specialist. I wasn't thinking that way. I was just glad to have the OK to see a proctologist. Things got worse for me at that point as now I had two crappy doctors telling me to suck it up and deal with it. The chronic pain had both a physical and an emotional effect. Finally, eighteen months after first complaining about my issue, my PCP sent me to a surgeon. My PCP made sure he got his shots in before sending me to the surgeon. He warned me that I would regret this decision. The surgeon, who was everything the other two doctors weren't, (i.e. competent, concerned, caring) took one look at me and asked if I was OK with him doing a biopsy.

"A biopsy; *who the hell biopsies a hemorrhoid?*"

You can fill in the blanks for yourself at this point. After the biopsy showed cancer, his nurse, who had assisted with the procedure, told my wife and me that the doctor knew this was cancer as soon as he looked at my anus.

Alright, it sounds to me like I'm whining and that's not my intention, but indulge me while I close the circle on this part of my first cancer journey. As I was still in an HMO, I had to go back to my PCP and get a referral to an oncologist and radiologist. When this jackass saw me, he shook my hand and told me how sorry he was about the cancer diagnosis. I reminded him that I had come to see him repeatedly over the past eighteen months, and he had done little about my condition.

His response, "Your problem is with the proctologist; not with me."

Yep, he was not only a bad doctor but an asshole to boot.

All of this was happening towards the end of 2006. The timing was fortunate as we were in our open enrollment period for benefits at work, which gave me the opportunity to opt out of an HMO program. It felt wonderful to dump my PCP and, better still, I ended up finding a great doctor.

Even though I am a self-proclaimed teller of tales, the story of life with these two bad doctors is the truth. I chose to bore you with this story because I wanted to drive home the point that having the right doctor is important. I don't think it's over dramatic to say that choosing the right doctor might be a life and death decision. I pretty much knew that my Primary Care Physician, when in the HMO, wasn't the best doctor in the world. The thing is, you can get away with having an OK doctor when you're relatively healthy. If you are only going to a doctor for an annual physical or for an occasional ache or pain, you may not need the best doctor in the world. The day that you have a serious medical issue is the day that you may regret having a moron for a doctor.

Look at it this way; let's say your mechanic isn't the best repairman in the neighborhood, but your car runs good, and you only take it to him for simple stuff like changing oil and rotating tires. That's fine until the day that your transmission starts clanking or your gears begin to grind.

I'm half Sicilian, and Sicilians use the word Omerta to describe a blood oath of honor. For example, a mobster, adhering to the code of Omerta, would violate the oath by testifying against another mobster. Omerta happens all around us every day. Like with cops; no matter how corrupt a cop might be, other cops would never drop a dime (snitch) on them. The scariest example of Omerta is in the medical profession. Doctors, knowing full well how bad some doctors are, will continue to not only protect an incompetent doctor, they will go on recommending them to their patients. Some of the fault lies with us, the patients. We assume that most doctors are competent. We assume further that they are intelligent since it takes brains to get through medical school. We are dazzled by the white coat and the stethoscope. The whole doctor package is meant to convey a sense of trust and confidence. The truth is, no matter what the profession, there are outstanding members in that profession and on the other end of the spectrum; there are people who are not very good at their job.

There's an old joke, "What do you call the guy who finished last in his class in medical school?"

Answer: "Doctor"

Doctors are not immune from incompetence and ineptitude just because they are well educated. No matter what profession or trade you look at you will find people who just suck at their jobs. I have never had someone say to me, "You know, I'm not too good at my job. As a matter of fact, I'm really pretty horrible at what I do. A monkey could probably do my job better than I do."

No one has ever said that to me, but there have been countless times in my life that I've encountered people who consistently do lousy work.

You may have a bad doctor if your doctor:
- Doesn't seem to hear what you are saying
- Isn't concerned about your concerns
- Lacks sympathy
- Says things that just don't seem right
- Is distracted during exams
- Is more worried about what kind of insurance you have than how you're feeling.

Being in my mid-sixties, I know a lot of cancer survivors and patients. An old friend of mine has melanoma, and he tells me his dermatologist always greets him with the same question, "What kind of insurance do you have?" He never thinks to ask my friend how he's feeling. This doesn't necessarily make the guy a bad doctor, but it does make him a Class 'A' tool.

•**KEEPS YOU WAITING**: (Please note that I took the time to write this in all capitals, made it bold, and then underlined it for greater emphasis).

Any doctor who can't adhere to a schedule, which they created for themselves by the way, is an inconsiderate a-hole. Let me get this straight…you're smart enough to get through med school but haven't unraveled the mysteries of how to use a clock. Alright everybody, take a step back here as I get on my soap box.

Dear Doctor, your time is not more important than my time. I have cancer, so no one's time is more important than my time. You keep me waiting each and every time I'm in your office because you don't care that I have to wait. You make no effort to fix the problem because you don't see it as a problem. How would you feel if it was your sick father who was left waiting for over an hour? Oh wait; you're an insensitive douche bag so you probably wouldn't care. Here's a sobering thought, doctors have a worse on-time record than your local cable TV operator. Let that sink in for a moment. How's that for a gut punch?

There have been several times in my life, after waiting for well over an hour for the doctor to grace me with his presence, that I have actually had the audacity to say something. They are prepared for this. I believe they take a class in medical school on how to handle the carbon blob in their office who dared to question 'Doctor'…not 'The Doctor'…just DOCTOR. The same way you would say God and not 'The God'. Doctors have been known to confuse themselves with eternal and omnipotent deities who created the heavens and the earth.

Here are some things I was told by a doctor after calling them out for being excessively late:

•*'I spend as much time with a patient as necessary. I would do the same for you'*. That may sound noble, but let's peel that onion back a bit. According to statistics that I found on-line, and let's face it, if it was on-line it must be true; doctors are late for appointments 50% of the time. What I see is a pattern: doctors, who are late, are late chronically. On the other end of the spectrum, doctors who are on time are usually on time consistently. The difference is one doctor sees punctuality as being important, and the other doctor is a self-absorbed, unfocused, disorganized butt-wad.

• *'Perhaps you would be more comfortable finding a new doctor'.* I have actually been told this by several doctors and hearing a doctor say this, after waiting over an hour, should be grounds for justifiable homicide. If you are a doctor reading this book, and you have ever in your life said this to a patient, you should do the world a favor and leave the medical profession. I believe the DMV is hiring; you'd fit in perfectly there. I can't fathom the arrogance it would take to say this to a patient.

The following is true, as if I would ever make anything up. I had an appointment with a doctor who was chronically and excessively late for every appointment I had ever had with him. As his office was in my neighborhood (10-minutes from the house), I called his office to ask if his appointments were running late that day.

"You want to know if DOCTOR is running late?" the woman asked me. She made no effort to hide the incredulousness in her voice.

"Yes, I live in the neighborhood and would rather wait at home instead of waiting in his office." To illustrate my naiveté, this seemed like a legitimate question to me. Sometimes I can be so stupid.

"What time is your appointment?"

I told her, and she said, "Then you need to be here at that time."

So, as a good patient, I showed up at the appointed hour, entered his packed office, and waited for well over an hour to see DOCTOR. I should not have had to call that day. If DOCTOR is running that far behind schedule, I should have received a call from his office telling me to come in later so I wouldn't have had to wait when I arrived that day. Wow, I can really say some stupid stuff sometimes, as if that would ever happen.

OK, I feel better now that I got that off my chest, and to all those doctors who do work hard to adhere to a schedule and try to see their patients on time, I apologize.

My primary care doctor over the past 12 years is amazing. It is very rare that I wait very long, if at all, in his office, and on the infrequent occasion that I do, he makes a point of apologizing. He's a great doctor and sadly, he's getting ready to retire. The message to all those other doctors is, *'See, it can be done'.*

So, how do you find a good doctor?

First of all, even if you are aware of a good doctor, you need to make sure they accept whatever insurance you have. Secondly, are they accepting new patients? Oftentimes, good doctors will not accept new patients for a variety of reasons. In the case of my doctor over the past 12-years (whose praises I sang above), he has been in practice for forty-years and has all the patients he can handle. If he was inclined, he could increase his client list without much difficulty. Bless him for not doing this as it might impact his punctuality as well as his level of care. News of a good doctor will spread quickly, and many will seek him out. If they really are a good doctor, they will set a limit on the number of patients under their care.

Urologists are particularly bad at growing their patient lists far beyond the point of what they can handle. Baby Boomers should just arbitrarily be assigned a urologist after reaching the age of fifty (provided they haven't needed one already). My first urologist, who came highly recommended and had excellent on-line reviews, was a horrible doctor. He sent me for a battery of tests and, weeks later, when I received no results; I called his office several times. When they finally admitted that they had lost the results, (but of course didn't apologize for the error) they suggested that I call the lab and see if they had the results. Yep, you heard that right; they wanted me to call the lab. I'm surprised this egomaniac didn't ask me to pick up his dry cleaning for him as well.

So, I found a new urologist, and I told him about my experience with the first urologist. He knew the guy. Of course he immediately told me how wonderful and competent and well-respected the first doctor was. Remember the code of Omerta...a doctor will never say something bad about another doctor. I asked this new urologist if he was a good doctor, and he assured me he was. I told him the problem was that there are a billion Baby Boomers out there and we're all pissing like racehorses, so he could be the worst urologist in the world and his waiting room would still be packed with people. This second guy was pretty good except that his waiting room was always packed, his patients always waited, and DOCTOR didn't seem too concerned about that part of his practice. This was the same guy whose office I was foolish enough to call to see if he was running late on appointments.

What about on-line review sites? Let me share a story. After years of going to my doctor, who, as I mentioned, is exceptional, I looked at his on-line reviews before going to visit him. I did this out of curiosity and whatever I saw or read wasn't going to change my high opinion of him. Several sites had him at close to five-stars, which is what I expected. One site, however, had him at three stars and this surprised me. There were only a few reviews on this site, so the one bad review weighed heavily. I broached the subject with him. He was aware of the site and the poor rating, the worst of which concerned his mishandling of a hospice case. My doctor doesn't manage hospice cases. All he could do was shrug it off as the bad review was meant for someone else. This doctor has a very common name. If you were to Google it, you would find a lot of doctors with the same name. He mentioned that there was even a doctor with the same name operating out of the same hospital along with my doctor, which, according to him, had the potential to create confusion.

Review sites are out there for everything from restaurants, to movies, and to doctors. I'll visit these sites before trying a new restaurant, and if the reviews are overwhelmingly weighted in one direction or another, it does influence my decision on whether or not to try it. In the case of restaurants, what I normally see is that for every one-star rating, there is a five-star rating to offset it, which doesn't really help in the decision making process.

Should you look at a doctor's on-line reviews when looking for a physician? Sure, why wouldn't you, as it represents another data source. If you hear good things about a doctor, but the on-line reviews are marginal, make an appointment and discuss it with him or her, or write them a note expressing your concern. A doctor's reaction to these inquiries might be a good indication of what that doctor might ultimately be like. If, to paraphrase the Bard, *"Methinks the Doctor doth protest too much,"* then you may want to keep looking for a new doctor.

Perhaps the best source for feedback on a potential doctor is what your family and friends say about them. Nobody is going to be more candid than a friend or family member. Count on them to give you the straight dope on a doctor.

OK, I'm going to get off this doctor thing now as I could write volumes on it, but keep in mind, as you get older, you typically won't get by with just having one doctor. Part of this has to do with us living in the world of medical specialization. The age of the simple country doctor who delivered babies, set broken bones, and tended to every imaginable ache and pain is a thing of the past.

Even though I've had cancer three times, I consider myself a relatively healthy guy. So by my delusional way of thinking, I'm pretty healthy, but the reality check comes when I start listing all my doctors. Besides my general practitioner, I have/had an oncologist, a radiologist, a urologist, a cardiologist, an ophthalmologist, a retina specialist, an audiologist, a physiatrist, a podiatrist, and a dentist. That seems like a lot of doctors for someone who describes himself as 'relatively' healthy. I could field an entire baseball team with all these white coats. That would be a good name for our team, 'The White Coats'.

I also have a veterinarian but that's for Abbey Road, our sort-of-a Black Lab. Abbey is prone to sympathy cancer as she had cancer along with me in 2018, and now in 2019, we are both going through cancer together again. How's that for a faithful canine companion?

Interlude Two: The Book I'd Never Write, Right?

Do you remember, back in my first Interlude, how I told you that my urologist was wrong and that there was no way cancer had found its way back to me so quickly? That was in the spring of 2019.

Dear Reader, we have just fast forwarded to June 10th, 2019. It's late at night, but I can't sleep. Today was my first day of chemo, well, sort of anyway, because as I mentioned, I have a lengthy history with cancer. Today was a long day. I'll go back again tomorrow to have more poison pumped into me and again on the following day. When I go back to chemoland tomorrow they'll want to know how I'm feeling. When they ask me how I slept, I'll tell them that I was up a lot during the night, which is unusual for me. They'll tell me that was a side effect of the powerful anti-nausea medicine they had given me. Maybe they should have mentioned this to me when they gave me the medicine, at least I would have known there was a reason that I was wired up and wide awake through much of the night. Maybe apathy was another side effect of the nausea medicine because I realize I'm not too concerned about the sleepless night.

I'm retired, and I start each day out by writing, so I normally don't care if I'm up for part of the night. It gives me a chance to think about the next day's writing. The novel I'm currently writing, 'Shade Tree', will be my fifth novel. I'm only about eight thousand words into it, but on this night, I'm not thinking about the minimum of five hundred words that I expect myself to write in the morning.

I'm thinking about cancer.

Today, I started my third battle with cancer, and as I lay in bed I find myself thinking about my history with cancer. It is getting to be a long history.

When I wake up, I will put 'Shade Tree' to the side and open up a new Word document and begin to write about my life with cancer. It's a book I never thought I'd write, but as the saying goes, '...and yet, here we are'. When I finish my writing session (never less than five-hundred words, as writers need to be disciplined) I am prompted to name the file. I call it 'CANCER BABBLE', which is fine for a working title and seems to fit the vague image of where I believe the book might be headed. As I close the document file after that first morning of writing, I can't help but wonder where this book is headed.

Will anyone even care about what I have to say?

Chapter Three-Cancer Round-One 2007

Courage...I encourage everyone who reads *CANCER BABBLE* to get to know a survivor, and I'll guarantee you'll hear amazing stories of courage and perseverance and fortitude and strength. Sadly, you won't hear any of these stories about me.

I'm not bragging when I say this, but I was not a very good patient. In retrospect, I could have been nicer. I could have been nicer to my family and my friends; I could have been nicer to my doctors and my nurses. I certainly could have been nicer to that woman in the hospital cafeteria. There was an incident, but in my defense, I saw that lime Jell-O first.

I was what the medical profession labels "a chronic whiner", which I later found out isn't even a real medical condition. At one point during my treatment, some so-called health care professional actually wrote that on my chart...

•Chris Drnaso

•6'-1" Caucasian

•Whiner...

I was such a pain in the_____, (I'll let you fill in the blank) to my oncology teams that they collectively called me in for what they said was a consultation. Of course you know you're in trouble when they tell you that you need to bring your mother. I told them my mom was dead, and now she's mad at me. My wife went with me, and when they got me behind closed doors they really let me have it. They described me as being difficult, rude, insensitive, petty, and unlikeable.

I am NOT petty.

Things really got out of hand when they threatened to pull the plug on me. My wife reminded them that I was not even on life support, to which they replied, "That won't be a problem."

OK, enough of that foolishness. In 2007, I went into my chemotherapy and radiation treatments with eyes wide shut. Nothing could have prepared me for the beating my body (not to mention my psyche and my emotions) were about to take. I was looking at thirty radiation treatments and close to 200 hours of chemotherapy. The chemo would be delivered via a pack that I carried around with me. It fed into a port that had been surgically implanted into my chest. Ain't that some space-age, Buck Rogers, shit? That was only a small part of this bizarre new world I now found myself being drawn into.

To give you an idea of how naïve (i.e. stupid) your author is, I fully expected to go through all of this standing on my head. Oh please; thirty radiation treatments; give me a break, don't you have something hard for me to do. Chemo, what is that, like Extra Strength Tylenol? No problem, I've got this. The main chemo that I was given at that time was called, and I'm not making this up, Five F-U. The emphasis was definitely on the F-U part of the name as in, "Hey cancer boy, I'm going to F-U up big time." Five F-U is still a go-to treatment for colorectal cancers and still guaranteed, as promised, to F-U up.

I was in excellent shape in 2005. That had changed pretty dramatically by 2007 when I went into treatment. I had lost weight and strength, but by far the worst damage two bad doctors had done to me over an eighteen month period was to my psyche and to my resolve. Emotionally, I was not in a good place at the beginning of 2007. That was the price I was paying for being under the care of Doctors Twiddle-Dee and Twiddle-Dumber, but we've been over that already, and I'm not going to chew that cabbage twice.

In 1998, long before my first cancer diagnosis, I entered an event called 'Hustle up the Hancock'. For those not familiar, the John Hancock building is a one-hundred story skyscraper here in Chicago. 'Hustle up the Hancock', is a fund raiser for the American Lung Association, and as the name implies, you walk up the stairs to the top floor of the building. I'm forty-five at the time, and if I may say, I'm in great shape for a guy in his mid-forties. I'm in the gym four or five times a week, lifting or taking aerobic or step classes. I'm competing against kids half my age in two-man beach volleyball tournaments. I am so ready for this, and can only think, 'Oh please;

climbing to the top of a 100-story, 1,128-foot supertall skyscraper; give me a break, don't you have something hard for me to do?'

I had not even reached the 10th floor before the reality of this challenge settled in. My legs are feeling it, and I'm sucking for air, and I still have ninety floors to go. I'm feeling each stair tread, and what I'm doing would not be described as 'hustling' up anything.

So, why am I dredging up this bit of ancient history? Because I approached my first round of cancer treatments with the same degree of naiveté that I took on the 'Hustle up the Hancock' challenge. Even though part of me was all too aware that on January 2nd, 2007, my first day of cancer treatment, I was not in the same shape as I had been in two years prior, I chose to ignore all the symptoms.

'There are none so brave as the completely clueless'. Do you like that saying? I just made that up. I walked into that chemo lab on the first day of treatment with the same bravado that I had when I walked up that first flight of stairs in the Hancock building.

For those of you who are wondering, I did make it to the top of the Hancock building on that spring day back in 1998, but the man who climbed that last flight of stairs was a much humbler person than the man who took that first step.

Thinking back to January 2007, and those first few weeks of treatment, I'm still overwhelmed at how quickly my resolve dissolved. The same way I hadn't gotten too far up the Hancock tower years earlier before the reality of what I had embarked on had set in.

I started both chemo and radiation in 2007 on January 2nd. (Happy New Year!) Less than two weeks later, with barely five radiation treatments and 100-hours of chemo in the books, I realized that I had sorely underestimated the brutality of this so called cure. The road to wellness, as it turns out, was a bumpy, pot-holed, road indeed. The radiation is starting to affect my skin. Early on, it's like having a sunburn; uncomfortable, but manageable. The chemo is zapping my strength. I'm tired, but not sure if it's the drugs or if I'm just losing the psychological battle. It's hard to be subjective about the fatigue. One reaction I'm dealing with, that is very real and very impacting, are mouth sores. I was unprepared for this, and by the time we actively began treating the sores, the damage was already done. Every part of my mouth and gums are tender, it is difficult to ingest anything. Solid foods are out of the question. I try protein shakes and supplements, like Boost and Ensure, but even sipping these are painful.

I mentioned that I had lost weight prior to starting treatment. I was convinced my rectal pain might be related to something I was eating, so for the year before I was finally diagnosed, I became very particular about what I ate and how much I ate. My misguided thinking was that if I ate less, I would have to evacuate less, as that painful part of my daily routine had become something to both fear and dread.

The perfect storm is brewing. I go into treatment below my normal weight and the mouth sores are preventing me from eating normally. My weight plummets. I am closing in on 160 lbs., and I regret the decision from decades earlier to throw away my clothes from high school.

Several weeks into the treatment, there is no question of subjectivity related to the way I feel. My fatigue has numbed me. Any activity, no matter how routine, exhausts me. My radiation treatments mark the passage of time. Like clockwork, Monday thru Friday, I show up at the radiation clinic, stick my buttocks into the air for all to see, and wait for the sinister looking machine to bombard me with something I can't see or hear but am starting to feel more and more with each treatment. What started out feeling like a minor case of sunburn has moved far beyond something marginally irritating or uncomfortable. My skin, throughout the entire rectal and genital area, is now burned as black as pitch. Let me repeat that, *'burned as black as pitch'*, lest you believe I misspoke or exaggerated. There is little that can prepare a person for what it's like to look down at your genitalia and see that it has been burned black. There is a scaly, reptilian look to the skin.

"What are they doing to me?" I ask myself. This can't possibly be the cure to anything. I reach out to another hospital and set up an appointment for consultation. I want someone else to look at this and tell me if this is normal. I meet with two of their oncologists, and guess what, they tell me this is exactly what they expected to see. Apparently, in the bizarre and

dystopian world of cancer treatment, having char-broiled skin is considered normal.

After twenty radiation treatments, a decision is made to give me a break and give the skin a chance to heal. I will still need to complete the last ten treatments, but for the moment I am glad for the respite even though I can't imagine how much healing will really take place during a two-week suspension of treatment. In truth, I can't picture a day when my skin will ever recover.

Is this the new normal for me?

The break in treatment, blessed as it may be, leaves me with more time to be alone with my own thoughts. My thoughts are dark; no one should be left alone with these thoughts.

I have forged a wonderful relationship with a Physician's Assistant (PA) who worked in my oncologist's office. During an office visit, even though it's difficult for me to talk about, I tell her I'm sad. Sad doesn't seem to be a strong enough word to describe all the emotions churning inside of me, but it will have to do as I begin to cry before I can say anything else. I am embarrassed by my tears.

There is an acronym, WWJD or 'What would Jesus do?' I grew up in the 1950s and perhaps a better expression would have been, WWJWD, or 'What would John Wayne do'? John Wayne, or 'The Duke' as he was commonly known, for those who have lived their lives under a rock, was the quintessential male role model through much of my life. John Wayne set an impossibly high standard by which a man should be judged. John Wayne would rub some dirt on it and get back in the game; he'd pull himself up by his boot laces and keep going, and most importantly, The Duke would never, ever cry.

I have forgotten every life lesson John Wayne has ever taught me as I am forced to admit that this whole thing is spinning away from me. It's easier for me to wrap my head around the physical beating I'm taking. I know these treatments are rough and that they take a toll on people. There's no big red 'S' on my chest, and I'm OK admitting to myself that I'm not Superman.

It's the emotional toll that it's taking that I was unprepared for. I'm in a doctor's office, in front of a virtual stranger, and I'm admitting to a weakness. I have been tested and found wanting. Worse than that, I'm crying. I could not possibly be acting more un-John Wayne like if I tried. I can picture the look of disappointment on The Duke's face.

"I'm sorry Duke; I am trying to be strong. I really am."

There are drugs that can help with this, the PA explains to me.

I graduated high school in 1971 and drugs were a big part of the counter-culture in the 60s and 70s. During that wild and wacky time, I believed that drugs might hold the key to enlightenment and held on to the hope that drugs would guide me to the answers to some of life's tougher questions. I experimented freely. I found no answers, and I came away having had more bad experiences with drugs than good. Not only that, whereas there were some people I knew from that time in my life that came away with an addiction to these drugs, that wasn't the case for me. Instead, I developed a healthy (unhealthy?) fear of drugs.

I accept the PA's prescription, and I go so far as to fill it. According to the Physician's Assistant, I would have to take this drug several times before it would start to have an effect. When the day came that I decided that I didn't need or want it anymore, it would take time for it to quit having an effect. I wasn't comfortable with that as I had seen too many instances where one never chooses to stop taking a drug. There are no shortages of stories about professional athletes who get strung out on painkillers. The similarity between those painkillers and the mood altering opiates I've been prescribed are too close for comfort. I own the drug, but I opt not to take the drug, but there is still a certain comfort in having it available. You know, just in case.

I cried a lot during February of 2007. It took almost nothing to get the water works going. One day, getting out of the shower, I took a good look at my legs, which had always been toned and strong from decades of sports and exercise. Now, at 160 pounds, forty pounds lighter than I was at the beginning of this nightmare, there is this big gap between my thighs. My calves no longer touched when I stood up straight. I don't know whose legs

I'm looking at, but these two spindly things can't possibly belong to me. If you think something like that wouldn't be a thing to cry about; you'd be wrong.

On one rare occasion, someone other than my wife took me to my radiation treatment. As we sat in the waiting room, this person decided it was a good time to tell me that I looked like shit. That's exactly how they worded it, "You know, you really look like shit."

When I made no reply, they decided that their assessment of me must not have sunk in, or perhaps I didn't hear, so they took it up a notch.

"I'm serious," they told me, "you look horrible."

It hurt to hear these words, my chin began to tremble, and I began to cry. Yep, I was sniffling like a baby right there in the waiting area.

"Have you been eating?" they asked me. "You have lost a lot of weight."

I fought the tears but cried harder. I didn't want to cry, but I couldn't help it.

"Your color's bad," they informed me.

That may have been the only day through all of treatment that I couldn't wait to get into the sanctuary of the radiation room.

In retrospect, I should have showed them my charbroiled testicles, and said, "You're worried about my weight loss, what do you think of this shit?"

Oddly enough, you will run into people on your cancer journeys who feel they are performing a public service by saying stuff like this to a cancer patient. I'm not entirely sure where this book is headed, but I am planning on writing a chapter entitled, *"Stupid Stuff People say to Cancer Patients"*. In fact, I look forward to writing that chapter as I have never met a cancer patient or caregiver that doesn't have a story that would fit nicely in that chapter.

Here's an important safety tip for those of you who might have interactions with cancer patients. We know we look like shit. How would we not know that? We see ourselves disintegrating every day? Do me a favor, if you get the urge to tell us how bad we look, don't. God bless the people who looked at my hair loss and my weight loss and the grey color of my complexion and said, *"Hey, you look good."* I would know that they were full-of-crap, but that was just fine with me.

I was amazed at how little it took to get me blubbering on most days. There were the ads with Sarah McLaughlin showing abused animals. Pass the tissues. I mentioned I watched a lot of M*A*S*H reruns and can't begin to tell you the number of times I got choked up while watching.

Sarah McLaughlin and M*A*S*H were nothing compared to the Marlo Thomas commercials showing those poor kids from St. Jude's Children's Hospital. Those little bald-headed cancer patients were guaranteed to have me sobbing each and every time I saw one of those commercials. To this day, those ads tug mightily at my heart strings.

As an aside, before I continue on my story, I want to close the book on my relationship with the Physician's Assistant that I mentioned above. My wife and I loved this woman. She was by nature a caring and concerned person, along with being a skilled health care provider. One day we went in for an appointment, and my wife and I got our first lesson in how difficult cancer is on everyone. We were told that she had left the practice, and when we asked why, we were told she just couldn't take all the sadness that goes along with working that closely with those afflicted with cancer. The things that made her so wonderful at her job; her caring and her compassion, were also what ultimately forced her out of that part of the medical arena. It takes a certain type to work with cancer day-in and day-out. Cancer is relentless and for every victory there are defeats. These professionals can't help but get attached to their patients as they see them so often during treatment. Sometimes these provider-patient relationships end by pumping the patients hand and wishing them a full and happy cancer free life. Other times, it ends when they attend their patient's funeral. There was a man who worked with my radiation oncology team from thirteen years ago that I still bump into occasionally. He never fails to give me a big hug and greet me like a long lost friend. Moments like those speak to the strength of the bonds that can be formed. I don't think I could do what they do, so God bless these professionals for their willingness to take ownership of this.

Sorry, I got distracted, but in a good way. Now let's get back to what's really important; talking about me. When last we left our tragic hero, he was fighting cancer for the first time. The year is 2007; he's being force-fed copious amounts of chemo drugs, and he's being bombarded with radiation from a space-age machine. Cancer has him against the ropes. He tries to fight back, but the beast is too strong, too determined. Each new blow zaps more of his strength; more of his resolve....

So what did I do?

Well, simply stated, I took it. I just took it. I didn't seem to have much of a choice. My radiation treatments started back up again. My skin, which I didn't believe could possibly look any worse, got worse. My fatigue, which I didn't think could be more crushing, collapsed upon me like a blanket of wet concrete. I wish at this point in the narrative I could tell you that I fought back; that I shook my fist to the heavens and declared that I had not yet begun to fight. There is nothing that I would like more than to tell you these things, but even though I am a story teller, I can't in good faith tell you that story. It's just too far from the truth. Your author, who had gone into treatment a scant two months earlier, believing he would be the poster child for all those dealing with cancer, is folding up like a cheap card table.

I'm wracking my brain trying to come up with a moment where I mustered my strength and struck a blow at cancer, but I'm coming up empty. Wait, does watching M*A*S*H reruns count? I watched a lot of M*A*S*H reruns; I still do to this day. I also watched a lot of the Australian Open in 2007. Serena Williams, who was unseeded going into the tournament, shocked the world by winning the women's title. As a writer, there's a wonderful opportunity here to tell you that Serena's battle to win against all odds inspired me to mount a counter-offensive against cancer, but that would be bullshit. You pretty much have to get up off the couch to fight back, and I wasn't inclined to do that on most days. Anyway, thank you Serena for giving a cancer patient something to cheer for during the cold and lonely winter days of January 2007. I have been a fan of yours throughout your illustrious career, and I for one was not surprised to see you win that major.

Day by day, I got closer to the finish line. I completed the last of my chemo-cocktails sometime in February. The following month, they bombarded my private parts with radiation for the last time. I was done. On the last day of treatment, my radiation team dressed me in a cap and gown, handed me a 'diploma', and snapped my picture. I cried at my 'graduation' ceremony; of course I did, but you probably knew that, didn't you?

Chapter Four-Caregivers

I talked about support earlier and how important it is for the treatment and psyche of a cancer patient. The key support element; the lynch pin that holds it all together when it comes to support, is the Caregiver. My wife, Marilyn, has been my caregiver through all three of my bouts with cancer. Her story is really very typical. She goes to bed one night with her husband and wakes up with a cancer patient, and by default, she's the caregiver. She gets no training, she has no experience, she didn't ask for the job, but none of that matters, as it's part of the wedding vows covered under the *'for better or for worse'* clause. A word of caution; you have to be careful with those wedding vows because you'll never know when they'll come back and bite you in the butt.

I always thought that being a teacher would be a pretty good job if you didn't have to be around those damn kids all day, and by the same token, the worst part of being a caregiver is having to deal with cancer patients.

This isn't to imply that all cancer patients are difficult to be around, but believe me, we have our moments. One might even go so far as to say that I had more of those moments than other cancer patients. I knew my wife had never applied for the caregiver job, but she stoically accepted the position without complaint. I understood all of that on an intellectual level but on another level, the one where I'm being a complete ass, I felt it was my responsibility to remind my wife that she had very little aptitude for this whole caregiving thing. Why would I do something like that? I just told you; I can be a complete ass. Please, pay attention.

So my wife not only finds herself in the caregiver role, she finds herself caregiving for a whiney complaining patient who thinks it's OK to point out faults with her caregiving abilities. Yep, I can be a real piece of work at times.

But through it all she was wonderful...very patient and loving and concerned. To illustrate, I'd like to share a story with you. I was napping one afternoon, and I woke up to find her fluffing my pillows. I was so touched by this simple act of kindness, and I knew she was trying her hardest to be the best caregiver she could be, and even though I knew I shouldn't say anything, I found fault with what she was doing, and I corrected her by saying, "No honey, the pillow's supposed to go behind my head."

I'm not stupid, and believe me, I found myself complaining a lot less after that little incident.

To my wife's credit, she realized pretty quickly that there was a complexity to being a good caregiver. She wanted to get better at it, so she went out and found a tutorial on caregiving. She was excited about finding the documentary and planned a whole *'Dinner and a Movie Night'* for just the two of us. So, she made us a nice little dinner. It was good, even though I don't think it's such a good idea to feed that many beans to a guy with anal cancer. You're pretty much just asking for trouble. After dinner, we sat down and watched the documentary together....it turned out to be the movie, *'Misery'*. She took notes, and kept saying things like, "This is good stuff; I'm learning a lot of good stuff here." To this day, I'm glad she never discovered the 'documentary', *'What Ever Happened to Baby Jane?'*

There might be a special place in heaven for caregivers. Perhaps a quiet corner with a sign reading:

"Caregivers Only!"
"No cancer patients allowed"

I think that would be a just reward for what some cancer patients put them through while on earth.

Cancer patients tend to be very busy people. You wouldn't think that was the case but those reading this book that have had cancer, know what I'm talking about. I was surprised by this when I went through it for the first time as from day-one I was continually on my way to appointments and treatments. There were labs, and blood work, and scans. It seemed like hardly a day went by that I wasn't scheduled to look at a white-coat somewhere for some reason.

It was rare that during this plethora of appointments, that my wife, my devoted caregiver, wasn't at my side. I can't begin to calculate the number of hours that she patiently sat in one waiting room after another while I was off somewhere getting pricked or probed or prodded. With only ancient magazines to keep her company, she sits, and she waits; stoically, quietly, faithfully. I fully expected to one day walk out of one of these sessions to find only a note pinned to an empty chair.

"Dear Chris, I love you," the note would read, *"But this is bullshit. P.S. Good Luck with this whole cancer thing."*

I wouldn't have blamed her for leaving that note, but she never did. After my treatment or my appointment, I would hold my breath as I peeked cautiously into the waiting room. I would breathe a sigh of relief to find her sitting there, with a magazine on her lap declaring that Dewey had defeated Truman. (The magazines were old; I'm not sure they were that old, but remember, I tend to make stuff up). She would welcome me with a smile. She'd then gather up *'The FILE',* and we'd be on our way.

A word about, *'The FILE'.*

As we were to discover, there is a lot of paperwork that goes along with being a cancer patient. Marilyn, my wife, my caregiver, and my best friend took charge of the paperwork. She started out with a folder, which we outgrew in no time. Next, she tried a binder, which was quickly replaced by an accordion file. This expanding file, being unwieldy, ended up in a book bag along with other cancer essentials. The barrage of paper was relentless and seemingly unending, and our fear was that if we stayed in treatment much longer, we would need a steamer trunk and a two-wheeler to haul it around from appointment to appointment.

The FILE went everywhere with us.

It became an extension of our very being.

We went so far as to name it.

We called it 'The Penske File' after an episode of Seinfeld.

Twelve years later, Marilyn still holds onto 'The Penske File'. I never asked her why she's kept all of this outdated paperwork. Perhaps it's just a silent reminder of a rough patch in our lives.

Through the whole ordeal, the cancer patient is going to get most of the attention. That makes sense, but the caregiver needs support, too. The same way they have support groups for the patient, many organizations cater to the support needs of the caregiver. If my wife should ever decide to attend one of these support groups, I hope the wine flows freely. I can't think of a group that deserves it more.

The cancer patient's job is to be sick; we have the easy part. The caregiver does most of the heavy lifting as they are expected to:

•Provide emotional support (even on days that they would like to strangle their cancer patient)

•Attend medical appointments

•Make difficult decisions

•Coordinate medical care, prescriptions, and schedules

•Provide transportation

•Manage finances

Perhaps the most difficult assignment for a caregiver is figuring out how to put on a smile every day, even on the days that there is little to smile about. They are the cheerleaders, and as such are expected to do the whole 'rah-rah' thing even when the home team is getting the tar beat out of them. The atmosphere surrounding a cancer patient can become toxic, and it's not healthy for a caregiver to breathe in that tainted air day-in and day-out.

As the cancer patient, I would receive cards and calls quite often from family and friends who were concerned with how I was doing. I don't remember a single instance when Marilyn received a card. It didn't seem strange to me at the time, but in retrospect it seems wrong and kind of sad. Many people would reach out to me to see if there was anything I needed. On most days, I didn't need anything. As the patient, I was being well taken care of.

My wife and I have always shared household duties. It is much more manageable when two people pitch in to do the yardwork, shopping, cleaning, laundry, cooking, etc. In 2007, during my first dance with the devil, months went by when I didn't raise a finger to help with any of that stuff. My wife and caregiver, on top of all the cancer related activities that get dumped in her lap, is now single handedly running the household. That makes for a very full plate.

If you are sincere about wanting to help the cancer patient, do this; the next time a friend or family member receives a cancer diagnosis, please reach out to the caregiver to see what they need. Be prepared as they will insist they need nothing, but offer the following anyway:

- Take the caregiver to lunch
- Take the patient for a treatment
- Sit with the patient
- Go shopping...either with or for the caregiver
- Run an errand
- Complete a weekly household chore...every week
- Prep a 'heat and serve' meal
- Send a card
- Take them out and get them shit-faced

All too often, caregivers are hesitant to leave their patients. The patient-caregiver link is a strong one. The two become one; their connection symbiotic. Their bond is a rich tapestry of dependencies and interdependencies. The welding of the patient-caregiver relationship, when forged in the fire of true love, is a beautiful thing to behold.

Chapter Five- Cancer Round-One Continued

In the spring of 2007, I completed chemotherapy and radiation treatments. I was declared cancer free. That's good, right? I knew I wasn't the same person that I was before treatment started, but that was OK. I was on the road to recovery. My hair would fill in; I would gain weight. I'm back, baby. Look out world, you are about to meet the new and improved me! Maybe not just yet, but soon, very soon, I'll be back to 100% normal.

Well, slow down there just a minute, Muchacho. It turns out that following thirty radiation treatments and two-hundred hours of chemo, normal tends to get redefined. What I recognized as business as usual prior to treatment may not be normal going forward.

The first indication that something was amiss was my lower left leg, which had ballooned to twice the size of my right leg. It looked silly, and I was worried that if this trend was to continue, I could end up looking like Popeye. Popeye may be a lovable American icon, but he's also horribly misshapen; I don't want to look like Popeye, not even in just one leg.

OK, so let's review. Over the past many months, I had been in the presence of multiple doctors multiple times. Not once during all of this face-to-face, white-coat time did any of these doctors think to say, "Oh, by the way, blood clots are a very common side effect of the cancer treatment you are receiving."

They never said that. If any of them had thought to share that important safety tip, I might have said, oh, I don't know, maybe something like, "That sounds bad, is there something I might do to prevent this?"

And, as it turns out, there were several things that could have been done proactively to reduce the risk of cancer related blood clots. But none of these preemptive things happened, because I was never told of the risk. The connection between cancer treatment and blood clots is not some well-guarded secret, known only to a select few doctors. This information isn't proprietary; you can GOOGLE it for gods-sake. It's common knowledge, but it's only valuable knowledge if this information is shared with the patient.

I'll be right back. I need to go back to the list that I labelled, 'You may have a bad doctor if your doctor...', and add, 'Doesn't fully explain all the consequences of what you are going through'.

My doctors, as mentioned, never brought up the risk of blood clots. If they had, they might have also told me that blood clots are extremely painful and debilitating. I did not know this, but I was about to find out first hand just how painful and debilitating these clots really were.

So, less than two-weeks after being declared cancer-free, I'm back in the hospital getting poked, prodded, and probed once again. (Let's throw in ultra-sounds and blood thinners this time for good measure).

Please allow me a quick rant about ultrasounds before I continue on. There is an awkward intimacy to having someone ultrasound your legs when looking for clots. They need to work that scanner device into some very private places. It would have helped a great deal if the young technician who was conducting the test had introduced herself and perhaps prepared me for what the test involved. Instead she chose to treat me like a slab of meat that had been unceremoniously dumped on her examining table.

Here's some unsolicited advice to health care professionals everywhere:

- Introduce yourself to the patient, ALWAYS, no matter why the patient has come to see you.
  - Ask if they understand what the test involves
  - If not, take a second to explain
  - If the test, like my ultrasound, involves working around Mr. Happy, please let the patient know that up front so they are not taken completely by surprise.

OK, I promised that would be a short rant, but one more thing before I move on. If your patient has wrinkles and grey hair, assume they may have some degree of hearing loss. Please, speak loudly and distinctly.

When a nurse or technician takes the time to do what I describe above, it makes the experience infinitely more pleasant. And seeing as how I'm not shy about speaking my mind let me add, I don't want to hear any bullshit about how busy you are. What I am describing above is integral to your job and just as important as every other part of your job.

OK, the rants over; let's move on. The blood clots have landed me back in the hospital again, but I don't want to be in the hospital; I want to get on with my life. I want to get back to 'normal', but I'm moving in the opposite direction of what I knew as normal.

Am I worried about the clots? Not really, but remember, I tend to be naïve and very, very stupid when it comes to the world of medicine. A clot doesn't sound all that bad, does it? It just means something's not flowing, you know, like constipation. Hell, I've had constipation before and it passes, so the clot should be no big deal.

Dear Reader, I was wrong. In fact, I could not have been more wrong about the long term effects of a blood clot. I really hoped that I might recapture some of my athleticism following the cancer, and I might have, but that was never going to happen following the damage done to my leg from the blood clot. Pre-cancer (i.e. pre-blood clot), I played volleyball, some basketball, and tennis. I've always loved playing freestyle and ultimate Frisbee. These are all activities that require quick starts and stops. You need to be able to jump. I couldn't trust my leg to do any of those things anymore. In fact, I couldn't trust my leg to make it through the night without waking me up to violent leg cramps. These leg cramps, as I was to find out, would plague me for years.

My intention in sharing the news about blood clots is not to play the 'Poor-Me' card. My goal is to educate. Knowledge is power, as the saying goes, and I hope that maybe I'll help at least one person avoid this same issue. As a final word, many years after developing the clot, I feel it still impacts my lifestyle on a daily basis. It is never good to have a major appendage that you can't trust to perform properly. (Oh grow up. I'm talking about my leg). That is some powerful juju.

Well, I guess as long as I brought up the 'E' word (i.e. education), I may as well continue on that theme. A little known fact is that when you go through cancer, you become the 'Cancer Answer Guy'. Weird but true, and I'm sure a lot of cancer patients and survivors and caregivers will understand that statement, as they, like me, are likely to be approached by people who want to know more about the cancer experience. Some will ask the 'Cancer Answer Guy' questions about treatment; sometimes their questions might be about doctors or screening. Sometimes, they don't know what to say to a cancer patient, so their questions might just be idle chatter to mask awkward silences.

There is a mystery surrounding cancer, perhaps because there are so many different types of cancer. The patient and caregiver might actually be a good resource for questions about their specific type of cancer, but every cancer is different; ergo, each treatment is unique as well.

One thing I discovered is that people are more likely to identify with a certain type of cancer if they can actually identify the afflicted body part. Take breast cancer for instance. Because people can readily identify breasts, they tend to be more sympathetic to those suffering from that infirmity. The same is true of lung cancer. Just about everyone could pick out lungs on a chart of the human body, and not only that, most understand what the lung's functions are. Anal cancer: most people can identify that part of the body, even though some people couldn't find it with both hands.

Oftentimes, we hear of a type of cancer, but we really don't know where that organ is located within the body, and not only that, we don't know the function that body part performs. Take pancreatic cancer for instance; we've all heard of it, but I'll wager that most people couldn't tell you where it is or what it does. I, for one, have no idea. I guess I could have looked it up and then pretended that I'm smarter than you, but I'm not only too lazy to do that, I'm not inclined to look up body parts because most of them are really icky.

What about Lymphoma? Maybe one in a hundred knows what the hell that is. Most people wouldn't know a lymphoma if it fell out of the sky and landed on them. What makes it even more confusing is that there are two types; Non-Hodgkin and Hodgkin's lymphoma. One of those is worse than the other, but in truth, I don't imagine anybody would want either one of them.

Which brings me to another important point; there is no such thing as a good cancer. Cancer sucks the Big Yazoo...that includes ALL cancers. Now, there are definitely some cancers that are worse than others but allow me to repeat; *there is no such thing as a good cancer*. Later in the book we are going to discuss stupid things that people say to cancer patients and many of these insensitive comments are related to the way people assess the seriousness of your type of cancer.

So, when I'm asked to play the role of the 'Cancer Answer Guy', by people who want to know more about living with cancer, I am very honest and very candid. I tell them that cancer is emotionally exhausting to the point of being physically painful. You feel cursed. You wonder why the universe has conspired against you, and you don't know what you have done to have these indignities rained down upon you. What you have to endure is humiliating, and all you can do is hope that tomorrow, or next week, or next year things will be better.

I can really sum it up for them by saying it's a lot like being a Detroit Lions fan. One difference is that when you are a cancer patient your hair just falls out. When you're a Lion's fan, you get so frustrated you end up yanking your hair out.

Full disclosure, I'm a lifelong Chicagoan who's married to a huge Chicago Cub's fan. Following my first bout of cancer my wife and I attended several Relay for Life events. The events typically invited a survivor in as a speaker, and invariably these speakers took the, *'nobody knows the trouble I've seen'* approach. I'm not judging anyone for their take on the cancer experience, but Marilyn and I tended to seek out the funny, inane, and bizarre side of cancer. When I approached her about the idea of writing a comedy routine about living with cancer, she was all for it. My wife has always been supportive, so I was not surprised when she embraced this notion. So, I wrote a routine and billed myself as the, *'The Cancer Comic'*. Marilyn not only supported the idea, she contributed to the content, which makes sense as I didn't go through cancer by myself; she went through it, too. In 2008 and 2009, I performed at multiple cancer fundraisers and events throughout northern Illinois. When I presented the material in front of the right crowd, which thank God was most of the time (but not always), it was special. It was therapeutic for me and wonderful to hear survivors and caregivers laughing. There were many 'screw-you-cancer' moments.

Anyway, I threw in this story about the Cancer Comic because back in the day, I did not use the Detroit Lions as the punchline to the joke. I, much to my lovely wife's chagrin, claimed that going through the agony and hopelessness of cancer was a lot like being a Cub's fan. Of course, the Cub's, after a scant 100 years, ruined that joke in 2016 when they won the World Series. Sorry Detroit Lions fans, it appears that Marilyn and her Cubs got the last laugh after all.

Chapter Six- The Quest for Normalcy

My quest for normal continued after my first battle with cancer in 2007. I went back to work. There is nothing like working to make a guy feel normal again. I've always been comfortable telling the world that I was 'The Cable Guy', but I spent most of my 35-year telecom career on the engineering side of the business. For most of those years I managed an engineering team. It was fast paced, which was perfect for someone who was trying to forget a rough time and get on with his life. I was 54 in 2007, so there were still more than a few years to go before I could think about retirement. In the words of Robert Frost, I had, 'Miles to go Before I Sleep'.

In time, friends, family, and coworkers quit treating me like a cancer patient. The sad look of concern on their faces as they asked me how I was doing slowly began to fade. Eventually, when they asked me how I was, it wasn't about the cancer anymore. It was more of a courtesy thing like, "Hey, how you doin'?" When someone asks 'how you're doing' as a courtesy, they're not all that concerned about your health; they're just being polite. That was good. Perhaps if they could forget about the cancer, maybe I could, too.

Marilyn worked at a local gym at that time. She was an aerobics instructor, and would also work the front desk. One day, shortly into my post-cancer recovery, she came home with news that the gym owner and his wife had very graciously offered me a free membership. I had always spent a lot of time in gyms. When I was younger, it was to play basketball. Later on it was volleyball. Beyond that there was weight lifting and group exercise classes. I was a gym-rat, and as a kid, I had the bad grades to prove it. Gyms had always been a comfortable place for me.

I remember walking into Marilyn's gym for the first time. It had been months since I had worked out, and for the past many, many months, I had done little besides sit on the couch. This was a new gym for me, but I did know the owners and a few of the members and some of the employees because of Marilyn working there.

I may not have known too many of them, but they all knew me, because they all knew Marilyn.

I was Marilyn's husband; the guy with cancer.

The people that I did know would approach me and cautiously ask how I was doing. Part of their hesitancy was because they just weren't sure what to say. Adding to the awkwardness was the fact that I looked like shit. I was really thin; I'm talking about an Auschwitz, Holocaust survivor kind of skinny. Completing the picture is my complexion, which is an intriguing lite-grey color.

Everyone is being very nice. People are typically nice to cancer patients and survivors. Why wouldn't they be? There's even one guy who I did not know who approached me and introduced himself. He said he had heard about my troubles, and he hoped I was feeling better. I realized that took courage for him to do that. We became friends. Others kept their distance. At any given moment, I might espy a member looking at me from a distance. They would break off eye contact immediately. Perhaps fear of contagion kept them from approaching me. Keep in mind, it's a gym; it's not a MENSA convention.

I was hoping being back in a gym would help me feel normal. It doesn't. It feels alien. I feel like an impostor. What am I doing here? I should be home on the couch watching M*A*S*H reruns. That's the only place that feels even remotely normal to me.

But I dragged myself to the gym, so I should at least try to work out. I get on the treadmill, which is a machine I am very familiar and comfortable with. Because I've used this machine so many times in my life, I know the speed and incline that I have always set it up at in the past. Today, that seems like a bad idea. *'Take it slow'*, I caution myself, and boy, did I ever. Ten minutes later, (and I'm not making that up; I might even be bragging a little when I say it was ten-minutes), I climbed off of the treadmill. My legs are shaky, and I worry about them supporting me. I didn't know you could make a treadmill go that slowly. If I had gone any slower, I might have actually gone back in time. I wanted to feel good about this first trip back to the gym, but I didn't. I found my way home, climbed onto the couch, and thought about my long road back to recovery; my road to normalcy. I saw it as a challenge, but in truth, I'm not really up for a challenge. I knew where I had been physically at one time not all that long ago and my trip to the gym showed me all too clearly where I was today. It was overwhelming to think of, and try as I might; I cannot envision a day when I'll be anywhere close to the shape I was once in. There are indeed, *'Miles to go Before I Sleep'.*

I did go back to the gym a second time, and then a third time and then on a regular basis. It started to feel more normal and less alien. My ten-minutes on the treadmill that first day slowly expanded to fifteen minutes and eventually to a half hour. It didn't happen that quickly, but it did happen. I started to fold some weightlifting into the mix. I took it slow; I took everything slowly. Because of the residual damage from the blood clot, I never did go back to the aerobics classes that I loved so much. The same was true of group sports like Ultimate Frisbee and volleyball. Tennis was in my wake as well. All of that was fine with me. I had survived cancer and was getting on with my life. I had no complaints. I went from being the cancer patient working out at the gym to just another guy working out. It felt normal and normal felt good.

When I first went back to work, I was on half days, which was good as those few hours were all I could handle. Most days I went home and slept following my shortened work day. Working and working out were therapeutic as were simple things like doing a load of laundry or running to the store. It's getting to be summertime and the grass needs to be cut and yardwork needs to be done. It takes me longer to do these things than it once did, but that's OK as I am doing them. I could feel the pendulum arcing back towards normal. It may be a new and yet to be defined normal, but it was still better than the cancer world I was leaving behind.

There came a day that my wife and I realized that we did not have another doctor's appointment for a month. This may not seem like a cause for celebration, but when you are in and out of clinics, labs, and doctor's offices several times a week, having a month off feels like winning the lottery. Happy days are (almost) here again.

Big companies love to reorganize. They live to reorganize. In fact, big companies focus so hard on reorganizing that some never get organized. Sometimes they are so engrossed in these reorganizations that they don't see what a disorganized mess they have become. In big companies, there is someone whose job it is to try to eliminate your job. It may help to picture this person as a grim reaper with a scythe in one hand and a spreadsheet in the other. That's how I envisioned this cretin. Never forget, in big business, at the end of the day, you are an expenditure on a spreadsheet; no more, no less. When you work for one of these big companies, you do so with the understanding that any day could be your last day. It doesn't make any difference if you are employee-of-the-year material or if you have a stack of stellar annual reviews. When a big company decides they can live without you as an expenditure to the bottom line; you're history. Hasta la bye-bye, baby.

Thank you Dear Reader for staying with me as I talked about big business, and I promise, I do have an agenda for telling you this story. There was a young man who worked for me at one time. He was an in-house employee who had lost his job several years before due to a reorganization. Almost literally, the day after he lost his job he was back at his same desk doing the same work he had done as an employee. The only difference was that one day he was an employee and the next day he was a contractor. This is a common practice with big businesses.

One day this young man stopped by my office and we got into a discussion about health care. He told me that he was on high blood pressure medicine. I was surprised as he was in good shape, and I knew him well enough to know he wasn't a drinker or a smoker. He went on to tell me that when he had lost his job during the reorganization, he discovered that he was considered uninsurable by many health care providers because of the high blood pressure.

That's when he hit me with the big tamale. He told me as a cancer survivor, I would also be considered uninsurable if I was to lose my job. This was a very sobering (i.e. scary) thought. I looked into it, and as it turns out, he was correct. Part of the equation was *if* I could find insurance, and the other part of this was; if I did find insurance, what would it cost? This was concerning as I worked for big business and, like just about everyone in the organization, I was anxious everyday about the possibility of losing my job.

I mentioned that Marilyn worked at the local gym at the time that I was coming out of cancer treatment. She liked the job; the owners and members treated her respectfully. Being a small, family owned business, they offered no options for insurance. That had never been a concern because she had been on my insurance for years.

I hated to do it, but I asked her if she would consider looking for a new job; one with benefits. She did, and we were blessed, as she found a job at the local school district as a teacher's aide. She was eligible for health care benefits with this job, but the irony is that she didn't take advantage of the benefit program as she ended up staying on my insurance. As a matter of fact, Marilyn was offered an annual stipend (bonus?) for NOT taking the insurance. If I was to lose my job, it would be considered a change in life status, and she would be able to sign up for benefits without having to wait for an open-enrollment period. As it turned out, this worked out great for us as Marilyn was able to forego her insurance and stay on as part of my benefits. Sometimes it's better to be lucky than good.

The thought of losing benefits, in many ways, is scarier than losing your job. Years later a bill called the Affordable Care Act (ACA) was passed into law. Depending on your political leanings, this was either the best thing that ever happened to the American public, or it was the worst. I can't comment on it as I never had to use it, and beyond that, I didn't read the act. If someone out there should actually read the thing, please drop me a note and explain it to me. The problem is that it's a long act. How long, you ask. As an aside, I wanted to tell you exactly how many pages were in the ACA. That sounds easy right. I went on-line and immediately got confused. No wonder those idiots in Washington can't get anything done, when they can't even agree on how many pages are contained in a piece of legislation. Hands across the aisle, my ass.

Health care in the United States today is complex and frightening and confusing. Our family has always been blessed with good health care benefits, but we have also lived in fear of losing those benefits one day. My heart goes out to those that do not have good health care coverage. I know this would have to keep you awake at night.

My apologies, perhaps I came on a little too 'gloom and doom' while talking about health care. There is a lot of talk about health care in this country and a lot of that discussion is centered on the high price of maintaining your health. Let's take a minute and look at it from a different perspective. Maybe there are ways to curtail some of these costs. People like to talk about thinking outside the box; so what say we think outside the health care box.

Let's start with a simple example, and I have to give my wife credit for this observation. We have a Dollar Store in our neighborhood, and let me say right off the bat that we have a 'real' dollar store. Everything is a buck or less. We don't go to those high end dollar stores where you might end up paying upwards of a $1.39 for some things. What? You think we're made of money? We're nobody's fools.

As we are leaving the store, my wife turns to me and asks, "Who would buy a pregnancy test from the dollar store?"

I had to admit, that was a stumper. The best answer I could come up with was, "I guess someone who's only mildly curious about whether or not they're pregnant."

So, if you're not all that worried about whether or not you're pregnant, your mindset might be, "Maybe I'm pregnant. Maybe I'm not. What the heck; it's a buck. I'll take the test."

If I can be very honest with you, for a buck, I'd be curious to take a pregnancy test, and I'm a sixty-six year old man. I'm sure I've blown a dollar on stupider things in my life.

I'm not here to judge the veracity and accuracy of a Dollar Store pregnancy test. My point is that it gives you the ability to perform a medical diagnostic test on yourself for very little money.

See, we're thinking outside the box.

When you think about it, there are multiple options for more cost effective medical care. Let's drive down the road a piece to the local Wal-Mart. They have a blood pressure machine right in the front of the store. What could be more convenient or a better value? There's a cuff for your upper arm so you can easily check your blood pressure, and there's also a spot for you to place your finger and it will tell you your heart rate. I use this machine often when I'm there. Well, I didn't use it last time because there was already someone using it. Not only that, but I had to tell the guy that the little slot was for his finger. It's hard to believe someone could get that confused, but it's a Wal-Mart, not a meeting of the Algonquin Round Table. An important safety tip: if you are at the blood pressure machine in Wal-Mart and you are unzipping your pants for any reason, you are doing something wrong.

I got a flu shot at Wal-Mart. It cost me ten-bucks, and not only that; they gave me a coupon for two-bucks off at the snack counter. That's a win-win in anybody's book. I hope I'm starting to make my point about affordable health care services.

I see a trend developing. There are already doctors working at Wal-Mart. Well, sort of; they're optometrists. But my point is they have opened the door to have more medical services available on site. Sears is way ahead of the curve on this one as you can go there to get your eyes checked, your teeth cleaned, and you can pick up a hearing aid while you're at it.

Let me ask you this; can the day be too far off from Wal-Mart having its own Cardiology or Oncology department?

Picture it, you walk up to the greeter, "Hi, and welcome to Wal-Mart," she says with a smile.

"Oncology, please."

"No problem darling," as she hands you a shopping cart for some unknown reason. "You can't miss it; just head towards housewares and make a left before you get to automotive."

Even though I can envision it happening, I'm not sure I'm ready for this just yet. Shopping at Wal-Mart is scary enough without hearing an announcement for, "Clean up in urology."

Interlude Three: It's only hair

July 4th, 2019. I am trying to walk you through my cancer life in chronological order. Even though the year is 2019 as I write this, I've been focused on telling you about my first go-around with cancer in 2007. Yesterday, July 4th, 2019, I lost my ponytail to cancer for the second time in my life. In chemoland, they told me I would not have a lot of hair loss. They were wrong. It started coming out by the fistfuls. There is little that can prepare a person for running a brush through your hair and seeing gobs of hair in the sink. It looked like a small furry animal was trying to make its escape down the drain. Looking at my pile of hair, I thought back to the musings of the comedian Gallagher when he asked, "What held it in yesterday?"

Losing your hair is sobering and a little sad. I asked Marilyn to cut it for me. I knew she didn't want to give me the haircut. Part of the reason was that my scalp was not only clearly visible; it was irritated, presumably from all the sudden hair loss. I sympathized with her reluctance, but I showed her that the *Caregiver Handbook* clearly states in chapter one that caregivers have to do a lot of shit that they'd rather not do. The ponytail was the easy part as it had been reduced to a few wispy strands. She cut the rest of my hair. It was emotional for her. We've been together since the early 1970s. We were hippies, and in many ways, we still are. In college, my hair cascaded down to the middle of my back; hers was down to her waist. She has always had beautiful hair, and I have always had hair. I guess I'm blessed to have kept my hair through 66 years, and many people over my lifetime would tell me that I was lucky to still have hair. Lucky? My hair has been grey and brittle for quite a while now. On windy days, I look like one of those popping party favors. I never thought of it as lucky or unlucky. It was just hair and I never really gave it a lot of thought. When Marilyn finished cutting, I looked at my new coif in the mirror. It's not a good haircut, but in fairness to my wife, I don't think Vidal Sassoon could have done much better. I now missed the days that I had looked like Professor Irwin Corey as now I had a striking resemblance to Gollum from the *Lord of the Ring* movies.

CANCER BABBLE

I lost a lot of hair from chemo in 2007 but that was nothing compared to this go-around. There's an old saying, *'you don't know what you got till it's gone'*, and the truthfulness of that old adage hit hard as I examined my bald head in the mirror. I became self-conscious and wore do-rags whenever I left the house. One day, while waiting for the light to turn green, I glanced over to a bus stop where three men were waiting. All three were every bit as bald as me, and as far as I know, none of them were in chemotherapy, and none seemed worried or even aware of their follicle challenges. In that moment, I realized that there were lots of bald men walking around. I just hadn't noticed. It should have been liberating to know that I, too, could discard my head wrap and join my bald brethren, but in the end, I couldn't bring myself to do it, and I continued to wear my bandanas.

A friend of mine, who had gone through breast cancer, documented her journey. She was a beautiful young woman with hair to die for. At one point during the process, she gave up trying to hold onto the last remnants of hair and opted to shave her head. She documented it all on film, and she wept as the trimmer swept its way back and forth across her head. Marilyn and I watched the video, and we both cried along with her. My heart goes out to all the women who have been faced with the same choice. In truth, it did hurt to lose my hair, but I can't begin to compare my chemo related baldness to the thousands of women who have lost their hair. Please don't accuse me of stereotyping, but a woman losing her hair is a whole different kettle of fish than when some old guy like me loses his hair.

Chapter Seven- Happy Days are Here Again or The Quest for Normalcy Derails

Sorry, I got distracted with healthcare coverage, and how to save on your medical bills, and then there was that whole thing about losing my hair. I'm back now, and I'm ready to take you through what I think of as my post-cancer 'salad' days. These were the years when I felt like I really put cancer behind me. At work, me as the cancer patient was becoming more and more of a distant memory, and people once again treated me just like they treated all the other worker drones. The same was true at the gym. Occasionally, a family member or friend would ask me how I was doing, and I knew they were asking about the cancer. I was happy to report that I was doing well and that cancer was behaving itself.

Each day made it a little easier to convince myself that the cancer was not only gone, but gone for good. And why wouldn't it be gone? Me, having cancer one time was a freak accident; a statistical anomaly. Surely, it would never happen again. I really believed that, and I believed it even more with each passing year. Plus, I had evidence that the rest of my life would be cancer free. My oncologist would send me for CT scans periodically and these scans showed nothing but good news. Not only that, but I started going for colonoscopies and that provided more good news. No polyps; no worries. Yep, it's all going my way.

Here's the thing about cancer; it doesn't play fair. It is a devious and untrustworthy opponent. On some level I knew this. I'm not a big fan of mirrors because of the way I now look later in life. My hair is grey and a lifetime of sun worshipping has creased my face with wrinkles. I'm gruesome, and mirrors drive home just how hideous I look. If I avoid mirrors, I can convince myself that my hair is still thick and black; my complexion taut. Being delusional is one of my better traits. I excel at it.

Because they own mirrors, cancer survivors are some of the bravest people I know, as every time they look at their reflection they can't help but wonder if this is the day their cancer will come back. But I didn't worry about any of that. Cancer had moved on in my life. It has gone off to bother someone else, and even though my heart went out to these new victims, I took comfort in the fact that I had battled the beast and won. Take that cancer, and in the immortal words of Rocky Balboa, *"You ain't so bad!"*

The salad days became months and finally extended to years. Our sons grew and left the nest as Marilyn and I started to think more and more about the day we could retire. Retirement held the promise of travel and adventure. These were wonderful things to look forward to. I was lulled into a sense of security.

There is an ongoing discussion amongst cancer professionals and researchers on whether or not we are better now at curing cancer or if we are just better at early detection and education. The medical community has embraced testing and screening. Women, in many cases from a relatively early age, are routinely sent for mammograms. If there are hereditary indicators that a woman might be predisposed to breast cancer, a good doctor will be even more diligent. Women proactively perform self-examinations. According to breastcancer.org survival rates for women diagnosed with breast cancer have tripled over the last sixty years. There are a lot of factors for this improvement including better medicines and improved surgical techniques, but a huge part of these kinds of statistical improvements has to do with education, screening, and early detection.

Early detection and screening is the key and might be the difference between you being a cancer survivor or a cancer fatality. Some of the screenings a person can do on their own, like a woman who routinely examines her breasts. This would be particularly important for a woman who has a history of breast cancer in her family, but in truth, it's important for every woman to develop this habit.

Everything I just said about women and breast cancer also applies to routinely checking your skin for any early signs of a melanoma. Do you have a sore that doesn't seem to want to heal? That could be a red flag. There are a lot of helpful web sites that detail what you should be aware of, and how best to examine yourself.

Another key component to early detection is having the right doctor. If you are concerned about something, and your doctor isn't, you may want to get a new doctor or at least a second opinion.

A work friend of mine, who was in his late-forties, mentioned to me one day that he was scheduled for a physical that afternoon. I was shocked when he told me that he had successfully avoided a prostate exam during these annual physicals. He went on to tell me that the doctor would get as far as getting out the rubber glove and the lubricant before my friend would tell his doctor that he was really not comfortable with going through with the test. The doctor would acquiesce. NOT COMFORTABLE? First of all, no one is comfortable getting a prostate exam; not the patient, not the doctor, not even you, my Dear Reader, is all that comfortable even reading about prostate exams. I told my friend that if he had a doctor that was not providing a prostate exam, he should seriously consider getting a new doctor. He laughed it off, and said, "Forget it, the next doctor might insist on doing the exam."

I've always been very proactive about my health. I've gone for annual physicals since I was in my thirties. When I turned forty, I asked my doctor about colon testing and prostate screening. When he told me I was too young, I told him that wasn't good enough. We compromised, and he ended up giving me what I called the *'shit on a shingle'* test. I'm pretty sure that's not the clinical name for the test, and I'm not sure if they still offer this test as I'm describing something from a quarter of a century ago. I'll describe how it worked and then apologize for being so yucky. I would poop and then smear a bit on a card. I'd mail the card in, and they would analyze it. Easy-peasy. I did this test a few times in my early forties. Truthfully, I was never 100% sure what they tested for; I was just glad to get a clean bill of health when the results came in.

I told my wife the same tired joke each year as I prepared to mail it out. Ready? "When the lab gets this, they are going to say, *'Look at what some asshole sent us'*." Cue the snare drum, thank you; I'll be here all week. Try the veal.

Screenings, typically, get more involved and in some cases more intrusive as you get older. Continuing on the theme of prostate exams, as I mentioned, it started with a mail-in test. Sometime around my mid-forties, when I went for my annual physical, there was the lube and the glove waiting for me. I was told we had graduated from the mail-in test and it was time to put a little more skin in the game. (Every pun intended). Yes, it's awkward and uncomfortable, but the good news is that it's over in less than a minute. Truth be told, my wife has described her mammograms, and I gotta tell you, those sound a hell-of-a lot more painful than the old rubber glove up the yazoo test. Neither test is anything a person would look forward to, but one must soldier through these indignities in the name of good health.

The rubber glove test is actually called a digital rectal exam (DRE). The doctor inserts his finger into your bunghole and feels around for anything that doesn't seem right. (i.e. enlargements, bumps or hard areas). Many men, and by that I mean apparently every man on the planet, begin to have peeing issues as they get older. These issues, like urgency, frequency, flow, dribbling, (that last one is something for all you youngsters to look forward to) are oftentimes related to changes in the prostate.

Before we move on, let me mention that if you really want to confuse the hell out of yourself, go on-line and read about prostate screening. There is a lot of conflicting information about when you should get tested, what kind of tests you should be going for, and even more concerning, what the results are actually telling you. I'm not here to help you unravel all of that, and in truth, I don't believe I'd even be able to clarify all of that even if I was inclined to.

There does, however, seem to be some absolute truths in all of this. If you have family members that have had prostate cancer, that's a RED flag. If you are an African American (please tell me that I'm using the politically correct way of saying that) with a history of prostate cancer in your family; that is a BRIGHT RED flag. I found the following statistic on-line and, in truth; I hope it's wrong as it is disturbing. The risk of prostate cancer in black men is about 60% higher than in white men. Another absolute truth is that if you hang around above ground long enough, you are going to have your prostate probed and prodded and analyzed.

So far, I walked you through the mail-in test and the rubber glove test. Are you done yet? Please, we're just getting started. If warranted by either hereditary factors or abnormalities felt during the rubber glove test, your doctor may send you for a blood test. The blood test is to measure your PSA or prostate-specific antigen, which is a protein produced by the prostate gland. As a young man, you would hang out with your buds and discuss numbers like earned run and batting averages. When men get into their sixties, it's more likely they'll talk about their PSA numbers. Ah, the joys of aging.

A low PSA number is better than a high PSA number. So, if you go for the blood test, and your PSA is low, you don't have prostate cancer, and conversely, if your PSA is high, you do have cancer. Well that was easy, except for this; there is **absolutely nothing true** in that last statement. Even though the PSA test is considered one of the best diagnostic tools for prostate issues; the results are open to a lot of interpretation. In fact, most men with high PSAs don't have prostate cancer. A high PSA might be due to a lot of different factors including an enlarged prostate gland, a prostate infection, recent sexual activity, and are you ready for this last one, a recent, long bike ride. I always knew that those torturous, rock hard bicycle seats were invented by some sick sadist, but now I find out that they can actually skew a medical exam. Who knew?

PSA testing straddles the line between being a good diagnostic tool and being unreliable. Statistically, about 25% of men with a high PSA have cancer. In an effort to muddy these waters as much as possible, I should mention that even amongst these 25%, there may not be much to worry about. Many of these cancers are of a slow growth variety and often don't move beyond the prostate, but if your PSA is higher than what is considered normal, there is a good chance that you will move on to the fourth leg of the prostate diagnostic stool, and that's a biopsy.

I mentioned earlier in the book that my first urologist was a moron. He was the one that lost my test results and then expected me to call the lab and see if I could get the results. What a putz. When I went to him, my PSA numbers were very marginally out of the normal range. He was quick to perform a biopsy. If I knew then what I know now, I would have fought him on that.

Did I think this guy was a bad doctor? Absolutely! (and an A-Hole to boot)

Did I think he was a bad doctor because he performed a biopsy? No, I don't.

Doctors live in a litigious world. They constantly need to be on guard against doing (or not doing) something that might land them in a courtroom. So, looking at it from his perspective, he has a patient that has a slightly elevated PSA, and even if he believes that the high PSA almost certainly does not indicate any serious issue, he's still going to send me for the biopsy. Doctors need to live by a CYA (Cover Your Ass) code. They need to make sure no one can find fault with their treatment, so that being the case, I had a biopsy.

A prostate biopsy is a serious and potentially dangerous procedure. Looking at the particulars of the test, it is done by poking a hole in your rectal wall to get to the prostate allowing for samples to be harvested. Your rectum is one of the nastiest places in the universe. Your colon is a bacterial freak show, but the good news is all of that nastiness is contained within the rectum; the bad news is that a prostate biopsy compromises that containment. I did not get an infection after my first biopsy. I did after my second one and it was pretty bad. I spent weeks on antibiotics including two mega doses that were shot into my buttocks. I was still luckier than a friend who spent a week in the hospital on an antibiotic IV following a prostate biopsy induced infection. In fairness to all, I don't remember a discussion about risks prior to the biopsy, but that is not to say that it was not discussed. I do recall after the second biopsy being told, *'if you don't feel well, give us a call'*, but I did not leave the office that day filled with any great sense of urgency. It felt like more of a boiler-plate thing they would say to all their patients.

Surveys show that even though there are risks involved in prostate biopsies, less than one-third of doctors discuss these risks with their patients. A third of doctors only discuss the benefits of a biopsy, and the last third don't waste their time by discussing either the pros or cons. I found these numbers on-line so please keep in mind the words of Mark Twain, that *'there are three kinds of lies: lies, damned lies, and statistics'.*

We're going to stick a pin in this last item about doctors who do and don't educate their patients about the risks associated with tests, procedures, and surgeries. Just to prepare you, when I do circle back to this discussion, I will most certainly be getting my rant on. I will most likely vent, and yes, there will probably be some childish name calling.

Once my PSA showed even the slightest elevation, I was given a prostate biopsy. The results were negative. Kudos to this doctor this time around, as he didn't lose the results of that test. He did however lose a patient, as I was quick to disengage from a doctor that I had lost all faith in. Truthfully, I didn't have a heck of a lot of faith in the guy to begin with. Trust me; he couldn't care less about losing a patient. Even bad urologists have packed waiting rooms. Let that truth sink in for a moment; scary, huh? Do the math: there are twenty billion baby-boomers out there, many of whom are peeing like there's no tomorrow. So, 'yes', you can be the worst urologist in the world and still have patients lined up around the block. There are times that I'll be guilty of repeating myself during this chronicle and this is one of those times. *If you think you have a bad doctor,* please*, go find yourself a new doctor.*

Even though, in retrospect, I don't think I should have had that first biopsy, I couldn't complain about the relief I felt at knowing my prostate was cancer free. But, here's the thing, once the mega-conglomerate, medical-industrial complex in this country becomes aware that there is an anomaly in a person's test results, they latch onto that person like a pit-bull onto a poodle. There was no escaping the fact that my PSA had tested above the norm, and in truth, there should have been concern. The PSA test, even with all the debate on its veracity, is still the go-to test for early detection of prostate cancer.

I'm a visual guy, and I pictured it like this, my name is on a spreadsheet and across the top of this spreadsheet are two columns. One column is labelled, 'PSA Good', and the other column is labelled, 'PSA Not Good'. My name is now in the 'not-good' column and that means I am in for continued PSA tests. I am in for a whole lifetime of PSA testing. I don't have a problem with this. It seems sensible, and it's just a blood test so it's not really that big of a deal.

I had to find a new urologist as my regular doctor wasn't able to order PSA tests. Evidently, the insurance companies expected that those tests be ordered by a urologist. So, I found a new urologist. I mentioned him earlier. He was good. It would have been even better if he knew how to use a clock and not keep his patients waiting so long. In addition, I liked the guy. Likability in a doctor is not only a good trait, it's also important to me.

I've been a stained glass artist for over forty years, and as it turned out, my new urologist started his college career thinking he would be an artist. Even though he switched his major, he still dedicated time to his artwork. So there was a common interest between the two of us. We probably could have gone out for coffee and talked for hours. Instead, when he would finally make it into the consultation room, after keeping me waiting an inordinate amount of time, he would settle in, and we would start to talk about all sorts of things including art. Even though I always enjoy talking with anyone interested in the arts, I would remind him, "We should probably move this along; I know you have people waiting." He would assure me we were fine and then go on like he had all day with nothing to do. Of course, I couldn't help but wonder if the reason I always had to wait for him was because he was *'shooting the shit'* with all of his other patients. I would feel guilty walking through his packed waiting room on my way out, even though I knew I wasn't the problem.

But, I did like the guy on a personal level and, more importantly, he instilled in me a feeling of confidence in him. I'll take that, as I've been a magnet for bad doctors throughout my life. If the opportunity arises, I'll tell you about the guy that did my vasectomy. If I was to give an award to the worst doctor I've ever been (mis)treated by, he would probably get the prize. I don't know for sure as I have had a lot of bad experiences. I don't know if I've just been unlucky in choosing medical professionals, or if there are just so many crappy doctors out there, that it becomes impossible to avoid them. I'm leaning towards the latter.

Now that my PSA was on the medical radar screen it did mean that it would be monitored and evaluated at regular intervals. This not only made sense to me; it seemed prudent and in keeping with my lifelong attitude about my health, *'If there's something wrong, I want to be the first one to know about it'*.

Chapter Eight-Nothing's All Bad

Hey there, Dear Reader, are you still with me? I just reread that last chapter and it bored the crap out of me, too. I know, *'Christ, is this guy ever going to shut up about his prostate?'* right; like it's the most fascinating thing in the world. If you also had trouble getting through it, you may want to do what I did and turn it into a drinking game. Read it again, but this time, every time I use the word 'prostate', you have to take a shot. The material won't get any more interesting, but you probably won't care after you toss back the first few.

We have spent a lot of time talking about the trials and tribulations of cancer, but you didn't need me to tell you that cancer sucks. That's pretty much an absolute truth, and if the statistic I made up earlier in the book is true, the one that cancer has affected close to 100% of the population in some way, shape, or form; then you already have first-hand knowledge that cancer is bad news.

Let's look at it as an axiom; if you are smart enough to buy this book, (and if you bought this book, then you are really smart!), then you are smart enough to know that cancer is bad, very-very bad, BUT, and this is a big but I'm throwing out here; is cancer all bad?

WHAT? Is cancer all bad? How could I possibly ask such a thing?

Promise me you won't toss this book into the garbage upon reading this next statement, but, 'No' cancer is not all bad. Nothing is all bad. Every cloud has a silver lining, April showers bring May flowers. Whatever doesn't kill you makes you stronger, and all that other crap.

OK, you don't believe me? Well, I guess the onus is now on me to back up that rather rash and bold statement.

Did you ever know someone who could 'out-sick' everyone in the room? I have a friend like that.

If...

- I have the sniffles
  - He has a cough
- I have a cough

- o He has a cold
- I have a cold
  - o He has the flu
- I have the flu
  - o He has pneumonia

That kind of medical one-upmanship would make me crazy, and I can't tell you how wonderful it felt on the day I walked up to him and said, "I got cancer; now, what have you got?" It's pretty hard to out-sick cancer. I'll tell you what; it shut him up real good.

Do you see where I'm going with this? Need more convincing? No problem.

I talked about my first battle with cancer at length, and even though it had some challenges, it was not all bad. I went through two-hundred hours of chemo therapy and thirty radiation treatments and there really wasn't much of a silver lining to either of those, but when I was through with treatment and on my way to recovering, I went to a Relay for Life event sponsored by the American Cancer Society and that's where the payoff came in… I got a free tee-shirt. Yep, 100% free, no strings attached. It really was a very nice tee-shirt but I was a little disappointed because I found out later that if I would have had two more radiation treatments, I could have gotten a free toaster.

OK, you probably figured out that I made up the thing about the toaster, but the fact remains that cancer can't be all bad, not when you're getting free tee-shirts.

And let's not forget about the cancer diet. I went from 'el-pudge-o' to heroin chic in three months. It was a lot more expensive than Jenny Craig, but you can't complain about the results. And who doesn't like to hear, "Hey, have you lost weight? You look good. I'm not crazy about what you've done with the hair, but you have really slimmed down."

Here's a quickie perk you can't argue with; over the years, I have saved a small fortune on shampoo and haircuts.

And then there's the Cancer Card. What, you may ask, are cancer cards? To people's credit, most are willing to jump in and help a cancer patient in any *small* way they can. Small is the optimum word in that last statement. I'll give you an example; when I was done with my cancer treatments back in 2007, the little hair I had left was a disaster. This was when I lost my ponytail to cancer the first time. I asked Marilyn to call her friend, who will do in-home haircuts, and ask if she'd be willing to come over and try to do something with what was left of my hair. My wife warned me that her friend was a very popular stylist, and she may be booked up for a while.

I told my wife, "Play the cancer card if you have to." Her friend was over within the hour. Now in fairness to my wife's friend, she is by nature a very nice and a very caring person...you can easily take advantage of that when playing a cancer card.

Yes, I realize I sound like a jerk, but there are times when a cancer card really comes in handy, and it's not only the cancer patient who benefits from the playing of a card. The person who extends the kindness towards the patient gets a feeling of warmth and satisfaction by helping in some small way.

So, when you really think about it, I'm actually doing them a favor.

I saved the ultimate *'Cancer's Not All Bad'* example for last and that's Medical Marijuana. There is a faction of the medical community that believes marijuana has medicinal benefits when dealing with cancer. At least that's what I think they said, I just smoked some really good shit, so I'm not sure if I really heard that or it's just the voices in my head again. Yes, there is research that supports the benefits of medical marijuana, but when I went to my doctor for a prescription, I was met with resistance. He had his reasons for his hesitancy, and he had some valid reasons for not wanting to write the script.

- He felt that more research needed to be done
- He didn't feel it was the best treatment option for me
- I had been cancer free for over three years at the time I asked for the prescription.

I whined, and he finally caved and wrote me the prescription, but I knew he wasn't happy about it. I tried to lighten the mood and asked if he could write me a script for a bag of potato chips to go along with the marijuana, you know, in case I get the munchies. He did not see the humor. Anyway, the timing couldn't have been better because I had tickets to a Grateful Dead concert that weekend.

The American Cancer Society offers a variety of services to cancer patients. They will help with everything from finding a ride to treatment to providing wigs to patients. The use of medical marijuana is now so prevalent that the American Cancer Society has come up with a whole new line of wigs. It's called their Bob Marley collection. Rasta Reggae, irie, irie, mon.

The marijuana landscape has changed a great deal over the last ten years. It's legal in some places and will probably be available everywhere in the next several years. This is mostly due to the idiots we elect to run things. I'm fighting the urge to launch into a political diatribe, but if I did, I would say that it would be nice to elect someone who could think of a way to fix issues while not destroying the fabric of this country. Legalizing marijuana and making gambling available on every street corner is an unhealthy solution to the issues that plague this country. I was in college in the early seventies. I was a hippie who probably smoked his weight in pot by the time I finally quit smoking that crap in my early thirties. Marijuana is a narcotic; legalizing it is dangerous and irresponsible and please spare me the argument about all the tax money that will be brought in as these same idiot politicos will just squander that money anyway... but that, like so much of this book, is just one simple man's opinion.

Like many other things, when I researched on-line about the benefits of medical marijuana, I ran into a lot of conflicting and contradictory information. It was confusing, and I came away with the understanding that medical marijuana lands somewhere between a great treatment option and a bad treatment option.

I do, however, believe there is a legitimate application for just about everything. If a person is stage-four terminal, and they believe marijuana will help them cope, then under those circumstances, I am all in favor of it. Hell, I'd give a stage-four terminal cancer patient heroin, cocaine, a carton of Marlboros, and a quart of Jack Daniels. I'd even throw in a hooker if they asked for it.

Cancer is not all bad. I know I'm repeating myself, but I warned you that I was apt to do that in this book. In this case, I did it because I wanted to cleanse the palette before moving on. There is some silliness in this chapter as I'm sure you figured out. Free-tee shirts and cancer cards don't magically turn cancer from a horrible experience into a good one, but I'm going to stick to my guns when I make the claim that cancer is not all bad.

Relationships with the people in your life, when you go through cancer, become better defined. Notice how I didn't say that relationships get better, but better defined. I am blessed to have a great marriage, but I'm not surprised. Marilyn and I met in 1973. We started out as friends and then realized pretty quickly that there was something more there. In forty-seven-plus years together, most of those spent as husband and wife, we have rarely had a cross word between us. We are blessed to have found each other, and I am so grateful and honored that such a wonderful and caring and beautiful woman would share her life with me. We are soul-mates and best friends, so it couldn't get any better, right? Marilyn has been by my side through three bouts with cancer. She has not only been my caregiver; she has been my biggest cheerleader. I love her deeply and it breaks my heart to put her through this, but it would be horrible and frightening to have gone through this without her at my side. Before cancer came into our lives, I didn't think our marriage could possibly get any stronger; I didn't believe our love for one another could be any greater.

I was wrong on both counts.

Cancer will test the mettle of your relationships in a blazing hot forge of angst, uncertainty, and conflicting emotions.

How's that for a heavy statement?

Not all relationships will fare that well when tested so mightily.

If your relationship can endure the ordeal of cancer, it will be even stronger than you ever thought possible. Sadly, where some relationships will bond ever tighter, others will unravel. It's hard being a cancer patient, and in some ways, it's even harder being a part of the support team.

When Marilyn and I welcomed our first son into the world in 1986, we were told that there might be some friends, ones who didn't have children, who would distance themselves from us.

We didn't believe that would happen.

We didn't understand why it would happen.

It happened.

Adding a child into a marriage and into a friendship can upset the balance of some relationships. The addition of a child or cancer into a relationship changes the dynamic of those relationships. There are countless instances where dad takes one look at his new born child, and says, "See ya!" and is never seen or heard from again. The same is true of a spouse who, upon discovering their husband or wife has cancer, also opts for a quick exit.

When I was diagnosed with cancer for the first time, we were again told that there would be some people who would distance themselves from us. They were right, as we felt some family and friends pull away. I had an easier time understanding this; just as I also understood that the dynamic of introducing a child into a relationship has similarities to introducing cancer into relationships.

It, at its core, represents change.

Change is stressful.

Even good changes in a person's life can be traumatic.

CANCER BABBLE

Cancer changes a person. The physical changes are obvious, but it's the more subtle changes that a person goes through that really conspire to reinvent a person.

I changed following my first bout with cancer in 2007, but it took me a while to realize that I was changing. I spoke earlier about the physical changes; the hair loss and the weight loss; the blood clot in my leg. I could see those things as well as anyone, and because each had some physical manifestation it was certainly easier to see, which in some ways made it easier to understand and to deal with. Perhaps I was so focused on these outward changes that I wasn't too aware of the changes that were happening to me the person.

Change how? I don't think anyone would ever describe me as a very serious person. As a matter of fact, the opposite is probably closer to the truth, but following my first dance with the devil, I did become more serious about things. Being diagnosed with cancer is like being slapped in the face with your own mortality. The idea that one day the sun would come up in a world in which I no longer existed is a very sobering thought. I blew the dust off of my bucket list and understood that I did not want to find myself at the end of life's path and realize, "Oh crap, the sand is running out of my hourglass, and I'm never going to get to half of the stuff on my list."

So, I changed. I took a more serious approach to life, because I realized it wasn't going to go on indefinitely. My new mantra became, 'No Regrets'. A college friend asked me one day if I'd want to go back and relive our college days. I thought about it briefly before I told him, 'no'. I had tasted life while in college. I had kissed a few girls and gotten into a few fights. I had cut myself a big slice of that life, and I had savored it fully. I had no regrets when I left the college life behind, and I knew I wanted to feel the same way when the final curtain fell on the last act of this drama that I call my life.

High on my priority list was to write a book. I've been an avid reader for my entire life, and I knew I wanted to write a book one day. So, I started writing a book, and soon realized that I was being consumed by the task, but not in a bad way. I not only wrote; I wrote with a passion. Never in my wildest imaginings did I believe that writing would ignite such a fire within me. Writing was just the first step on my mission to make sure I would leave this world with no regrets.

This was the new me and I discovered that I liked the new me. I was proud of the fact that I was more productive and more focused, but as it turns out, the new me didn't set well with some people. There were friends that wanted the same goofball that they had known for decades. They were more comfortable with that traditional version of me. They wanted Chris Classic. They missed the card; the cut-up, but that guy was becoming more of a memory each day. I didn't ask to lose their friendship, the same way I didn't ask for the cancer. I didn't orchestrate the change; I just changed. I expected them to understand this metamorphosis and accept the new me. Instead of trying to understand and accept that cancer is a life changing event, they greeted me with pettiness and intolerance. They dispatched me with extreme prejudice.

I'd like to tell you I didn't care.

I'd like to tell you I was better off without them.

That wouldn't be true.

Losing friends hurt; pure and simple.

They hurt me.

Growing up, there was a kid in the neighborhood who broke his leg the first week of summer vacation. (That's not one of Dante's Circles of Hell, but it should be) This kid, who played baseball with us every day and rode bikes with us, suddenly couldn't do any of those things. He was on the sidelines; life had benched him. My mom would ask me to go visit him and sit with him, and I would promise that I would. I didn't. The kid was damaged goods. I went out of my way to avoid walking past his house. I considered it an inconvenience to have to do that. I thought about him less every day until I didn't think about him at all. When his leg finally healed, he came back into the fold, but we both knew that things would never be the same between us again.

Decades later, following cancer, I realized that, to some friends, I was now damaged goods, and they avoided me like I avoided the kid with the

64

broken leg. That karma train had circled back and slammed into me pretty hard.

At other times the alienation isn't as well defined as a broken leg. Friends just simply quit calling. It's not like getting a pink slip in your last paycheck. At least that would serve as a distinct point of termination. Friendships, exposed to the intense glare of cancer, become like a Polaroid that has been left out in the sun. Each day the photograph becomes less distinct. The print yellows and the edges curl. There comes a day when you discard the picture as whatever meaning it once had is now lost. It simply faded away.

Christ, I can be a maudlin bastard at times. Here I start out jokin' and tokin' about the upside of cancer and somehow I end up telling you about how cancer can implode your relationships. OK, let's see if we can put a different wrinkle on this before we move on.

Cancer, like life itself, is a journey. Some journeys are special, like when my dad drove the whole family to California one summer to visit our aunt and uncle. There were five of us crammed into a midsize sedan. We didn't have a lot growing up; five of us shared a one-bedroom apartment. There's a picture of my two sisters and me sitting on the rickety back steps of the apartment building. Years later, I said to my sister that the place looked like a tenement. She told me that was because it was a tenement. Who knew?

Our car was old; probably too old to trust it to make it to the west coast and back. There was no air conditioning. The interstate system was still being built, which meant we spent a lot of time crawling along on secondary and tertiary roads. We ate most of our meals in cheap roadside diners and spent nights in places that looked way too much like the Bates Motel. Pops was in a bad mood for most of the trip, and who could blame him, as he had to put up with my sisters and me. He wasn't a young man at the time (I was only eight and he was already in his mid-sixties), and he was exhausted at the end of each day as he was saddled with all the driving as our mother didn't drive. Thank the Lord, my mom never learned to drive. God bless her, but at four-feet-ten she would never have been able to reach the pedals or see over the steering wheel. All I can envision is her driving us over the edge of the Grand Canyon.

So for two weeks I was either bored, or hot, or fighting with my sisters for an extra inch of space in the car, or getting yelled at, but you know what, as miserable as that trip sounds in retrospect, it will always hold a magical place in my memories.

I think I'd describe my cancer journeys the same way.

Chapter Nine-You haven't heard the last from my prostate

Dear Reader, I know at this point you are saying, "Please, get back to your prostate issues. It's not fair for you to keep us hanging on like this!" OK, you're probably not saying that, but part of my purpose in writing this book is to walk you through my multiple inspirational and heroic battles with cancer. Yes, I used the words inspirational and heroic. I told you, as a writer, I'm inclined to make stuff up.

So when we left off, I was telling you that my PSA numbers were out of the norm and that I had found a new urologist and this new guy was going to take over the job of monitoring these PSA numbers. Do I really need a doctor to do this? Wal-Mart, if you're out there listening to this, is there a chance you can put a PSA testing station in your stores? You can slide it in right next to your blood pressure machine. I know I can come across as an idiot sometimes, but I'm serious about this. Why do I need to go and wait in my urologist's office for him to see me? The PSA test spits out a number and that number is either a good number or a bad number. Wal-Mart can have a little chart next to the testing station describing where your PSA number lands across this spectrum. If the number is in the good range, then I grab a cart and complete my shopping. If the number falls within the bad range; I'll go see my urologist.

The reality is that Wal-Mart does not have a PSA testing station...yet. Trust me, the day will come when they will, but until the dawn of that enlightened day, I will continue to go see my urologist. And that's what I did for several reasons. One, I felt it was important and prudent to continue to monitor these results, and secondly, as I mentioned earlier, *'If there's something wrong, I want to be the first one to know about it'*.

My new urologist not only monitored my prostate PSA levels, he also managed my BPH or Benign Prostatic Hyperplasia. "What the hell is that?" you may ask. I'm not sure, but if you have BPH issues it means you are peeing a lot, and in my case, I was peeing morning, noon, and night. I hope it doesn't sound like I'm bragging, but if there was an Olympic Urination Team;

I would have made the squad. I might have been named the captain of the team. When you have BPH you either have to pee, just finished peeing, or are looking for the next nearest bathroom as you know you will need to pee again soon. BPH is often related to an enlarged prostate, which was probably not the case with me. At the time, a friend mentioned that his urologist had prescribed Cialis (yes, that Cialis) to help control his BPH. I was intrigued, and asked my urologist about it on my next visit. That was one time I didn't mind waiting in his office. It was true. Cialis, most commonly used to treat E.D. or erectile dysfunction, had been approved as an effective drug to use for BPH issues. Not only that, Lilly, the manufacturer, was offering a 30-day free trial prescription. (Try it, you'll like it!) So, I filled the prescription, and I can honestly say it didn't do a goddamn thing for my BPH. I was still pissing like a racehorse every chance I had, but you know what, I didn't care. This wonderful magical drug had recaptured and resuscitated my libido from when I was a teenager. It was like being sixteen again. Just so you know, these BPH issues had nothing to do with my cancer, so you are probably wondering why I would even include this in my book. Did you really think I would walk around with a boner for thirty-days and *NOT* tell you about it?

Whenever my urologist performed the DRE (digital rectal exam) he never felt anything out of the ordinary which was encouraging. Over a period of close to two years, he monitored my PSA and that's where the trouble came in. I mentioned earlier, for those of you who are paying attention, that just looking at a PSA result only tells part of the story. The numbers are open to a lot of interpretation. Anyway, in early 2016, my PSA numbers were hovering above ten, and that is a number that no urologist is going to ignore. He performed a biopsy, and because of my PSA numbers, I couldn't argue with the wisdom of having this second biopsy. It was following this biopsy that I had the bad infection. When the biopsy procedure was complete, I asked him if he thought the results would show cancer. I could have kissed him when he said that he was almost positive that there would be no cancer. I believe he based this on the fact that he never felt any abnormalities when performing the rubber glove test.

Sadly, he guessed wrong, and the results of the biopsy came back showing cancer.

What to do?

What to do?

What to do?

As I was about to find out, that was going to be a difficult question to answer.

Because of all the radiation I had been exposed to while going through anal cancer, there was a question of whether radiation treatment would even be an option for this newly diagnosed prostate cancer. I met with a radiation oncologist who told me I would be a terrible candidate for any more radiation. He did however push to have the cancerous cells that had been captured during my biopsy sent to a lab that does a 'deep-dive' examination of the cancer. Prostate cancer comes in a variety of flavors and colors, and some of these cancers are more likely to live contentedly within the confines of the prostate, and cause little grief to the patient.

I'll get right to the good news; my prostate cancer, upon intense scrutiny, was not considered aggressive. Unfortunately, if I was able to handle more radiation, I would have been a great candidate for radiation therapy, but alas, it was not meant to be.

Chemotherapy? Technically there is no chemo treatment for prostate therapy, BUT (another big but) if the cancer moves out of the prostate, (metastasizes), chemo becomes an option. By my way of thinking, if the cancer moves out of the prostate, it's no longer prostate cancer, but what do I know?

There are three standard approaches to prostate cancer; monitor it; radiate it; remove it.

In my case radiation wasn't an option. Not only that, but the radiation I had received in 2007 left a concerning amount of scar tissue in the area of the prostate. (Cancer treatment....the gift that keeps on giving) When discussing a surgical solution, excessive scar tissue becomes an issue as it is not inclined to heal like normal skin would. Prostate surgery after radiation becomes a lot more difficult and there are many surgeons who aren't interested in performing this tricky procedure.

Tricky how, you may ask. If a surgeon is too aggressive in removing the prostate, there is a chance he will damage the bladder or the rectum. Damage to those vital body parts increases the chance of post-surgical incontinence. Wait, it gets better. A prostatectomy (prostate removal) following radiation could leave the patient with a colostomy bag. If a surgeon is not aggressive enough, and stays too far away from the bladder and rectum, he runs the risk of leaving some prostate tissue behind. This tissue is most likely to contain cancer, since it is in these regions that most cancers arise.

This doesn't put me in a good way.

To recap; radiation is not an option for me, and I'm a horrible candidate for surgery.

My urologist sent me to someone he considered the best in Chicago at dealing with these tricky kinds of issues. This urologist/surgeon/oncologist said, "Radiation is not an option for you, and you are a horrible candidate for surgery."

Well, I certainly feel better now that we cleared that up.

The only good news in this is that my cancer had tested out as being a slow growth variety, so I didn't have to do anything immediately. It was decided that I would go into a period of what was called 'active observation'. This seemed to make the most short-term sense. Just like it sounds, I would go to my urologist every couple of months, and they would monitor my PSA numbers. I had no choice, I had to go to him, as Wal-Mart still hadn't put in a PSA testing station; thank you very much.

So, for probably about the next two years, I dutifully went to see my urologist to get my prostate checked. The numbers would 'yo-yo' up and down, and of course, my sincere hope was that I would have to do nothing about my troublesome prostate for the rest of my life. I'm good at doing nothing; I really am.

In late September of 2017, my PSA number came in at 16.2. Even though there is a hopeless amount of contradictory and confusing information about the validity and usefulness of PSA numbers, the reality is that a number like 16.2 is going to turn some heads.

Before I move on, I wanted to mention that if you can manage to stay vertical in this world for long enough, the medical community quits worrying about things like PSA numbers and prostate issues. It's true. When you pass the age of about seventy, and you haven't had any concerning prostate issues, the medical mindset becomes that old age or something else is going to do you in long before your prostate. I guess that's good news. I certainly would have looked at it that way if I had made it to seventy without any issues. It didn't work out that way for me; I sincerely hope you have better luck.

My urology specialist sent me for another biopsy and an MRI. This was right around Christmas of 2017. Because it was the holidays, and because I had gotten a pretty serious infection following my second biopsy, I asked the biopsy doctor if he could mega-dose me with antibiotics. The doctor performing the biopsy actually thanked me for mentioning this and then went on to shoot an additional dose of strong antibiotics into my buttocks. Kudos to this doctor for not only listening to his patient, but for believing that a patient might actually have important information to share about his health. I did not get an infection this time around and ended up having a very nice and non-eventful, non-infectious Christmas and New Year's.

At around the same time, I went for an MRI (Magnetic Resonance Imaging). An MRI is a non-invasive imaging technology that uses strong magnets and radio waves to produce three dimensional detailed anatomical images. Boy, did I just sound really smart there or what? Actually, it was a definition I found on-line. This would be my first MRI, but I did know a little bit about MRI testing from friends who had gone through the procedure, so I was not surprised when the doctor asked me if I was claustrophobic. He said he would prescribe something for me to take on the day of the test to take the edge off. Since my free-wheeling, drug-taking days of the early 70s, I haven't been inclined to take anything stronger than a Tylenol. I told him I didn't think I had issues with claustrophobia and turned down the prescription. Later that day, I had second thoughts about it, so I called his office and told him I had changed my mind and would like to have a little something-something on hand just in case I was feeling overwhelmed on the day of the test.

My test was scheduled for 6:00-PM on a Sunday night, which seemed odd. Hospitals are a 24-7-365 business but when I arrived at the hospital that night, with my trusty caregiver at my side, we were both struck by the otherworldliness of walking into a huge medical facility that was both dark and empty. We fully expected a security guard to stop us and tell us we must be mistaken and that the hospital was closed. You need to leave; there's nobody here but us chickens. It wasn't a mistake. Marilyn and I were led deeper and deeper into the recesses of the hospital. We passed offices, all of which were abandoned and corridors that led to unlit and unknowable places.

I eagerly gobbled down the pill; thankful that I had asked for it. I was sorry I didn't have one to offer Marilyn as she looked like she could use it, and she wasn't even getting a test. I kissed her goodbye and left her to sit alone in a large, dimly lit, and completely empty waiting room. I was anxious about leaving her to fend for herself in such an alien environment. I glanced over my shoulder at her as I was ushered off to meet my MRI fate. Her smile didn't hide her angst as I could see the worry on her face.

A friend of mine has a history of back problems and has had quite a few MRIs over the years. I know it is very stressful for him, but he tends to be dramatic about things, so when he described what it's like, I would discount much of what he would say about the test. I owe him an apology as there are few things that are more bizarre than an MRI.

First off, I now fully understood why my doctor had asked me if I was claustrophobic. Once you are positioned on a table you are slid into what might be described as a new age sarcophagus. I went in with a plan, albeit a simple plan, for the claustrophobia. Are you ready for it? I wasn't going to open my eyes throughout the entire test, with the thought that what I can't see can't hurt me. I had asked how long the test would take, and I was told it would be approximately forty-minutes. They lied. An hour and fifteen minutes later the test finally ended, but let's not get ahead of ourselves. I swear to you, Dear Reader, that I did not so much as twitch an eyebrow during the entire length of the test. I barely breathed. Can a person hold their breath for seventy-five minutes? I think I did. The technician administering the test can talk to you through headphones, and twice this sadistic bastard informed me that I needed to stop moving around so much. Move around? Michelangelo's 'David' moves around more in the course of a day than I did during that test.

My plan of keeping my eyes closed was working really well until I foolishly opened them. It was just for a nanosecond but that was enough. Well, I found out something about myself that day; I do have claustrophobic leanings. There was perhaps an inch of clearance between the tip of my nose and the walls of the coffin I was laying in. I snapped my eyes closed but it was too late as I had glimpsed the wall of the tomb that enclosed me. I tried to un-see what I had just seen. Even through closed eyelids, I could feel the tightness closing in around me. At the beginning of the test, they place a call button in your hand. It was really a panic button. I was not going to press that button. As much as I hated that machine, and as much as I wanted this test to be over, I was not going to press that button.

Going into the MRI, I knew about the suffocating environment the machine creates. That's pretty much common knowledge. As I was getting prepped for the test, the technician offered me headphones and asked what kind of music I'd like to listen to. That sounded like a great idea, and I told him I liked smooth jazz. Smooth jazz sounded just about perfect to put me in a mellow state of mind. OK Chris, you took your happy pill, now just keep your eyes closed and listen to some music and this will be over before you know it. I love it when a plan comes together.

Now here's something I did not know about an MRI test. They are loud. Let me reemphasize that last statement. They are really **<u>LOUD!!!</u>** I was not prepared for this, and the first sounds the scanner made sounded like the fire alarm going off. I fully expected the technician to rush in and tell me we needed to vacate the building. Noises that the MRI machines produce have been compared to jackhammers, alien spacecraft landing, clanging, banging, and the sound of heavy industry going on in the background. Perhaps it would help if I told you to picture a blacksmith working at his forge... six inches away from your head.

Are there reasons the test needs to be so loud? I'm sure there are, and I'm sure some techno-geek could probably explain those reasons to the patient, but you know what? I didn't want to know the reasons. What I wanted to do was find the Doctor Frankenstein who had created this torture device, duct-tape him to a gurney, prop his eyes open ala *A Clockwork Orange,* and slide him into this hideous machine of his own invention. Give me a second to bask in the joy of that glorious image....ahhhh.

And what about the Happy Pill I took? The exam was over, and I was home for several hours before the damn thing kicked in. Timing, as they say, is everything.

Sorry, I got carried away remembering my MRI. There are times I'm easily distracted. It's time that I bottom-line this, and the bottom-line is that the results of this latest biopsy and the MRI are not good. My hopes to do nothing about my prostate cancer are dashed. Regardless of whether I'm a good candidate for surgery or not, there will be a surgery in my future.

Crap!

Chapter Ten-Are you out there, Lord?

"People say there are no atheists in foxholes. A lot of people think this is a good argument against atheism. Personally, I think it's a much better argument against foxholes."
Kurt Vonnegut

I hope you liked the Kurt Vonnegut quote. I was glad to have the opportunity to include it as he's a brilliant writer and will always be one of my favorite authors. My guess is that most of you have heard the expression, "There are no atheists in a fox hole?" The words 'fox hole' can be substituted for a multitude of dire or frightening situations or surroundings. For instance, you might say there are no atheists on the Space Shuttle, or there are no atheists riding the 'L' late at night in Chicago. At one time, I would have written, *'There are no atheists at Wrigley Field'*, but I can't say that anymore because they won a World Series. I'm a lifelong Chicagoan, who loves all things Chicago, and I'm married to a die-hard CUBS fan, but that doesn't change the fact that when the CUBS won the World Series, they ruined a lot of good jokes for a lot of comedians.

In France, during World War One, much of the fighting was done from trenches, and by all accounts it was a terrifying experience. It is generally believed that's where this 'atheist' saying came from originally, but like everything else, if you look it up on-line there are differing opinions on its origins. During the war, men would hunker down in serpentine trenches that branched out for long ways in multiple directions. A short distance away, across what was commonly called 'No Man's Land', the enemy sat in trenches of their own. Day in and day out, the soldiers on both sides of no-man's-land would sit in these dank, disease ridden holes and hope the next bullet didn't pierce their helmet, or that a mortar wouldn't fall from the sky and land on top of them. As these soldiers sat in their little hidey-holes, their thoughts were consumed with everything from the imminent threat of death hanging over their heads, to the fact that their saturated shoes and wet feet might lead to trench foot, and then to gangrene, and ultimately to amputation. The archival pictures of these soldiers, thousands of miles from home, lost in thoughts of Sunday dinners with the family and girls they left behind still make for powerful and haunting images 100 years later.

Cancer is like that. It, too, is a terrifying experience. Perhaps, we could edit this saying one more time to read, *'There are no atheists in a cancer ward'*. Many cancer patients will get closer to their faith, or their religion, or their God when going through cancer. I was like that...it happened to me.

Allow me to share a story with you. I was in chemoland one afternoon, and as I sat there, I prayed the Rosary, which is something that gives me a sense of peace and comfort. Patients come and go in chemoland as people start and finish their treatments at different times. A gentleman was led in and I watched as the nurses prepared to pump poison into this recently arrived patient. I mentioned that I'm a lifelong Chicagoan who loves all things Chicago, and of course, this includes 'Da Bears', so I couldn't help but notice that this new patient was a Green Bay Packers fan. I knew this because he had this little lapel pin attached to his hospital smock and on the pin was the Packer logo. Allow me to mention that the Green Bay Packer's logo is the letter 'G'. Really Wisconsin, the best idea you could come up with for a logo was the letter 'G'?

Moving on, in addition to the lapel pin, he was wearing this big chunk of cheese made out of some kind of yellow foam rubber on his head. I guess by his way of thinking walking around with a fake cheese hat on your head was somehow better than being bald.

Anyway, the 'cheese-head' and I struck up a conversation, and even though we were hardwired to dislike one another, that did not happen. It turned out that he was a very nice man and that we had a lot in common. We liked a lot of the same books, movies, and food and I thought to myself; *for as crazy as cancer is, it can also break down so many barriers*. It ended up being a very nice way to spend the afternoon as the time went by quickly. Cancer can be exhausting, so I was not surprised when my new Packer fan friend started nodding off to sleep. I went back to my Rosary, but before I did, I looked up to Heaven and said a prayer of petition and thanksgiving.

"Lord, you've blessed me with so much. I have a wonderful wife, two great sons, a loving family and amazing friends, and I want you to know that I love every minute that you have given me here on your green earth, but Lord there's so much left that I want to do before you call me home, so please, if there's any room for negotiation here... take the Packer fan."

Sorry, you caught me making shit up again, as there was no Packer fan in chemoland that day, but other than that, there was a lot of truth to what I just wrote. Philosophers have looked for proof of the existence of God since the beginning of time. I guess I'm one of the lucky ones as I see proof every day that God is in our world and in our lives. Keep in mind that I'm a dumbass and don't have nearly as much grey matter as the world's great thinkers, but that doesn't alter the fact that God is very real in my universe. He has blessed us with an Eden to live in, complete with pristine snowfalls, breathtaking sunsets, majestic mountains, and a panorama of colors to dazzle and amaze us every autumn.

How could you not find God in these wonders?

The fact that man is hell-bent on polluting this paradise and blowing this planet to smithereens isn't God's doing; these tendencies for self-destruction fall squarely on man's shoulders. We have every opportunity to embrace one another, but all too often, we choose to shun each other instead. God has given us the ability to create symphonies, but we use our talents to build bigger bombs. When given the choice between loving and hating one another, we opt for hatred. If man put one-tenth of the effort he puts into war into making a better world, we would live in an incredible utopia. We are the only thing that stands in the way of making this dream a reality.

There's an old joke about a man who is on his way to an important meeting. As he drives, he gets more and more stressed out because he can't find a parking space. He's going to be late if he doesn't find a place to park soon.

Desperate, he looks to heaven and prayers, "Lord, if you help me find a parking space, I swear I will go to church every Sunday for the rest of my life."

At that very moment, a car pulls out of a parking place right in front of him.

As he maneuvers his car into the space, he looks once again to heaven and says, "Never mind, Lord, I just found one."

Yes, I realize I got off on a tangent there, so let me circle back to my original thought. When life is going along swimmingly, you may not feel any strong compulsion to actively look for God. I had God in my life long before I was ever diagnosed with cancer. When cancer hijacked me, I never thought about blaming God. Instead, I reached out to Him (or Her, if you prefer) and asked that He stay even closer to my side as I went through this challenge. I have rules for praying and one of those rules is to ask God to grant me what I need the most. I leave what that might be in His hands, as I believe He knows what's best for me. I thought about this a lot in 2007 while going through cancer for the first time. I knew that people died from anal cancer (most notably Farrah Fawcett) and, of course, I hoped I wouldn't be one of those people. Did I pray at the time for God to spare me from that fate? No, I didn't. I asked the Lord, through prayer, to guide my life to whatever the best possible outcome was for me.

Maybe my attitude towards prayer has less to do with religious philosophy and more to do with some embedded ideas about prayer that I've carried with me since childhood. Some of the ideas we adopt as children and bring with us into adulthood run the gamut from weird, to funny, to just plain stupid. I've always believed that prayer is a tricky thing. I know this makes no sense, but I tend to look at it the same way I look at the genie in a lamp. We all know the way that works. You find a lamp, you rub it (yeah, that's real normal), and a genie appears. The genie offers you three wishes. Now I know that prayer has nothing to do with genies or magic lamps or wishes, but these off-centered ideas are what I carried with me from when I was kid. In case you haven't figured it out; I wasn't all that bright as a child.

So, you find the magic lamp and you get your three wishes, and of course, you wish for a butt-load of money. Now this is the tricky part; where does the money come from? Maybe you get hit by a car driven by some rich drunk guy, and you sue the bastard, and you get oodles of money in the settlement, but here's the kicker; you're in a wheelchair for the rest of your life. Ain't that some messed up shit?

That pretty much explains why I'm cautious with how I pray and what I pray for. The upside to having an attitude like this towards prayer is that whatever happens, you assume God measured and weighed your situation and has acted with your best interest at heart.

I'm going through my third battle with cancer as I write this, and of course, I hope I make it. If I don't, and if God does call me home, it's because that's what's best for me. There is a lot of comfort when you buy into that point of view.

Let's get back to the genie for a moment. Let's say you don't wish for a bunch of money; let's say you wish for a long life. That sounds good, right? Who wouldn't like a long life, but that wish is ripe with paradoxes. We had a close family member who lived into his early nineties. He was blessed to have had many more good days than bad. One very typical New Year's Day, he was at our house drinking beer and eating beef sandwiches while we watched football. A month later we buried him. If you're going to pray for a long life, that might be the life you want to pray for.

On the other end of that spectrum is our neighbor's wife. She was always a bright, attractive, professional woman. When we hadn't seen her for a while, and by a while I mean several years, word came to us that her dementia had gotten so bad that she was placed in a care center. My guess is she was in her early eighties. I believed the Christian thing to do was to pay her a visit. It wasn't a good visit. I didn't even recognize her when I saw her, and of course, she had no idea who I was even though I had been her neighbor for over thirty years. Her frailty and her vacuous stare haunted me as I drove away from the facility.

Did I pray on the way home? You bet your butt I did. I prayed for this woman. I prayed that God would do what was best for her, while I believed right down to my very core that the best thing He could do for her would be to call her home and back into His eternal flock.

Did my prayers end there? No, they did not. I may have broken my rule that day on my ride home by asking God for something more than just Him acting in my best interest. I prayed with all my heart that He might spare me from that same fate.

Pray for a long life if you wish, but pray with caution, lest God hear you and grant you your wish.

There is, in my humble opinion, too much concern with what religion a person is. I was raised a Catholic, but truth be told, I'm not a very good Catholic. I like to think of myself as a Christian, but I've been around so many Christians in my life who have such myopic views towards God and their fellow man that I hesitate to align myself with that lot. There was a radio DJ on the air here in Chicago at one time who had a whole collection of different on-air personas that he would perform. One of these characters was his 'Born Again Christian' whose catchphrase was, "Hi, I'm a born again Christian, and I hate you." I would laugh when he said this, but I also saw the truth in it. I have known many people who had found Jesus, which should have been a good thing, except for the fact that they immediately began acting in the most un-Christ like ways imaginable.

What's up with that?

Christians believe you are totally screwed in the afterlife if you have not accepted Jesus Christ as the one true Savior. If you believe that, then that's fine, but you need to believe it with your whole body and soul. If you are going to talk that talk, you better be willing to walk the walk. I've always thought that was a stupid expression but believe it actually works in this context.

My heaven is welcoming of anyone who has led a good life here on earth, which I know flies in the face of traditional Christian beliefs. I have no problem with sharing my heaven with Buddhists and Hindus and Muslims. I don't know what Heaven looks like. I think it might be different for everyone depending on how a person envisions the afterlife. If you think Heaven is people floating around on clouds and playing harps, then who am I to tell you you're wrong. I realized a long time ago that going to church religiously (Yep, that's a pun) every Sunday, was not going to punch my ticket through the Pearly Gates. I mentioned that I take comfort in the Rosary. When I say the Rosary; I say the Our Father, which is a beautiful prayer. The Our Father contains the line, '...*forgive us our trespasses as we forgive those who trespass against us'*. If I say the Our Father hundreds of times a year, and thousands of times in my lifetime, but I'm an intolerant prick who isn't inclined to forgive anyone's trespasses, then I should save my breath. Words mean nothing, it is what's in your heart that makes the difference, so if you go to church every Sunday and pray the Our Father, but have turned your back on a friend because of pettiness and intolerance, then good luck getting into your own Heaven. I know if I was guilty of these same thoughts and deeds and actions, I wouldn't be accepted into the version of heaven I envision for myself. That's the kicker within my philosophy; I am ultimately the one who decides what my afterlife will be like. That being the case, I step through this life very cautiously each day.

My views of religion and God are pretty much of my own design, and I've made my peace with that. If you asked me what God looks like, I wouldn't have a good answer for you. When I was a kid, God was typically portrayed as a kindly grandfather type. If it helps you to think of Him that way, go right ahead. I was never too concerned with how he looks as it never seemed important. Paradoxically, I have looked upon the face of God many times in my life. I see Him in the joy of children at play. He's present in the wrinkles of the aged. Look for him whenever one person stoops to help a fellow man. When someone fights an injustice in the world; He is there.

But, closer to home, Marilyn and I arrive at chemoland. It might not seem like a bad place to spend the afternoon as I get to sit in a comfortable recliner. There's a TV and snacks available. I read or nap or do crosswords while Marilyn crochets baby blankets for needy children. The chemo nurses are really nice. The reality of where I'm at and why I'm there sets in as the needle slides in and the chemo drugs begin to course their way through my body. I am comforted in the knowledge that He is at my side because, '*There are no atheists in a cancer ward*'.

Interlude Four: My Eulogy

July 29th, 2019: Today was my first day of round three of my chemo treatments. Like the first two times, treatment started with strong doses of anti-nausea medicine and, as in the past, these meds kept me up during the night. Cancer patients are continually being told to keep a positive attitude. I understand that, but there are times, especially when lying awake during the night that my thoughts are as dark as the room I lay in.

In truth, my bedroom is never entirely dark during the night. I sleep with a nightlight on out of necessity. We share our home with Abbey Road, a large Black Lab who we love dearly. If we turn off all the lights, Abbey becomes a Ninja dog. She is invisible in the dark, coupled with the fact that she might decide to lay down anywhere, makes her a potential death trap. Abbey has an Indian name; InDaWay because she is always in-the-way. A dark room, combined with a black dog that delights in getting in the way, is a recipe for disaster. If you met Abbey, you would like her; she's very sweet, but if you should come to our home take heed; she has an impish sinister side to her and seems to have an innate sense for getting under your feet. After having tripped over her several hundred times, I'm convinced it's no accident. I'll have to keep my eye on her.

Back to the night of July, 29th. As I lay in the *semi*-darkness, my mind wanders to everything from the ridiculous to the profound to the disturbing. I realize that Marilyn and I have yet to have the difficult conversation about the future. By this I mean the ultimate future. I believe we share the thought that if we ignore the tougher issues, the more uncomfortable questions, perhaps they will just go away. For example, as I lay here, I am worried, not for the first time, that we have never purchased burial plots. We have never even discussed it. Might it be that if I don't make arrangements for the end, then the end won't come? Of course, in the light of a new morning, that thought will seem silly and superstitious, but in the quiet darkness of my room at 2 o'clock in the morning, the thought has a certain importance to it. It not only seems important, it somehow seems urgent.

This cancer is different from the others. It was diagnosed as small cell carcinoma, which is considered both rare and aggressive in bladder cancers. Rare and aggressive; could you possibly come up with two scarier words when it comes to cancer? I promise myself that I will look into burial plots and arrangements at first light, but I will break that promise. I'm either a coward or just lazy. It's easier to think of myself as lazy.

At some point in the darkness, I realize that I've begun writing my eulogy. This should seem strange to me but it doesn't; it seems right somehow. I believe that funeral eulogies, like wedding toasts, are both important (and hopefully not delivered at the same event) but all too often they are not good. The best man is usually drunk, unprepared, or worse yet, believes he can just 'wing-it'. Yep, we have all suffered through those toasts.

With eulogies, you typically don't have to worry about the person delivering the eulogy being drunk unless it's the priest or if it's someone from my wife's Irish side of the family who has passed away. I realize that my eulogy is too important to leave in just anybody's hands. I will need to take ownership of this first thing in the morning. Like with the purchase of the burial plots, it is a commitment that I do not follow through on. Once again, I'm either a coward or just lazy. This time I'm pretty sure it's not laziness.

On my third day of my third round of chemo, I'm not feeling well. It's not the chemo; it's something else. After 24-hours, I realize I've caught a cold. Normally, a cold is no big deal but it is definitely impacting me as it hits right on the heels of the chemo treatments. One of my favorite movies is *Fiddler on the Roof.* In one scene, Tevye, the Jewish milkman and central character, is hurrying home on the Sabbath when his horse comes up lame. As he harnesses himself to his milk wagon, and struggles towards home with the sun quickly setting, he looks to heaven and asks God, *"Was this really necessary?"*

I feel that way about the cold.

Chapter Eleven: It's only Prostate Surgery

It's only prostate surgery. That's the way I looked at it. Prostate issues and subsequent surgeries had seemed so commonplace by the time I was diagnosed that it felt like you couldn't swing a dead cat without hitting someone with prostate issues. By my way of thinking, if these surgeries are so routine, then they are no big deal. In my lifetime, I had seen so many medical procedures that had gone from being painful, scary, and intrusive to being commonplace. This, to my feeble, uninformed, and delusional mind, included prostate surgery. Christ, I can be so naïve (stupid) about things.

When I was in high school, in the late sixties, if one of my sports heroes hurt his knee and needed surgery it was a very big deal. The player would have his knee laid open and would end up with huge Frankenstein monster scars that crisscrossed the joint. Recovery took a long time, and the patient either continued to have issues or, worse yet, the knee would fail him again (sometimes quickly).

Fast forward to the age of arthroscopic surgery. In this procedure tiny incisions are made and an even smaller camera (an arthroscope) is inserted into the affected area. From that point, it becomes more like a video game than a real surgery. A large monitor displays what the camera is seeing and the doctor lets the video guide his actions. Depending on the procedure, if the patient isn't out cold, he can actually watch the surgery. The day may come when there's a concession stand right there in the operating room where the patient can stock up on popcorn and Milk-Duds before settling in and watching their very own surgery. When I go for a colonoscopy, they give me what is called a 'twilight' drug, which may or may not knock a person out. The doctor will typically offer me the opportunity to watch. What kind of sick perverted bastard would want to watch their own colonoscopy? It's never really an option for me anyway as the twilight drug knocks me out cold. Thank God for that. Just wake me when it's over.

When I think about it, given this new world of arthroscopic surgery, it would be important for me to know that my surgeon is good at video games. I believe that it would instill a certain confidence in me knowing that my doctor had the high score at Asteroids while in medical school. It would show me that he had good dexterity and hand-eye coordination. A surgeon should have a Pac-Man game right there in his office. If I can beat him, then maybe I don't want him doing my surgery. If he sucks at PONG, do you really want him messing around with major organs? Asteroids, Pac-Man, and PONG; I guess you can tell I haven't played video games for a long time. If you saw me playing any of those games, you wouldn't be impressed, and you certainly wouldn't want me doing your arthroscopic surgery either.

Up to this point, I have been talking about advances in knee surgeries and described the procedures as arthroscopic surgery because it had to do with a joint in the body. The other side of the same coin is known as laparoscopic surgery, a term used with minimally invasive organ related surgeries. I hope I'm correct about that. I'm not a doctor; I'm not even very good at video games, but I read up about these procedures on-line, and I think I have it right.

So, for several reasons, I approach my prostate removal (prostatectomy) like it's going to be a cakewalk. For starters, it was described as 'minimally invasive'. If something is being called 'minimally invasive', it can't possibly be that bad, right? Secondly, and I touched on this earlier, I considered it a common surgery. You can't be in your sixties and not know people who had prostate issues. You would need a score card to keep track of all the people getting their prostate removed. Even more encouraging, I'm not going to funerals for men who have died from prostate cancer. I mentioned earlier that there are no good cancers, but prostate cancer seems less dangerous and deadly than other cancers. Some people I knew were treated with radiation and others had to have the gland removed. I knew one of my favorite singer-songwriters, Dan Fogelberg, had passed away in his mid-fifties from prostate cancer but that was surely an anomaly. Successfully surviving prostate issues was all about early detection and screening, and I would give myself five-star reviews in both of these categories. Yep, this is going to be a cake walk.

But, let's get back to the actual surgery. It's minimally invasive and commonly performed, both of which lulled me into a deeper world of delusion. In addition, it's laparoscopic, which means a couple of small cuts and wham-bam we're done. Say it with me: C-A-K-E-W-A-L-K.

I mentioned earlier in the book that I was going to get my rant on over doctors who do a bad job of patient education. The time, Dear Reader, to explore that subject is now upon us. Even though my doctor/urologist/surgeon/oncologist had a reputation for being one of the best in all of Chicago, he did little to nothing to prepare me for this surgery.

For starters, I found out after the fact that a prostatectomy is considered a major surgery. I had no idea. I thought it was more like a root canal; something that nobody would volunteer for but still not that big of a deal. There is a Medicare requirement that says I have to go see my regular doctor within a week or two of the surgery. I wasn't sure why I was expected to do this, but when I went; my doctor told me that this was some sort of a 'hand-off' consultation. (Don't hold me to that terminology. It was called something like that). I'll mention this again as he deserves it; I love my regular doctor. He's bright, knowledgeable, and punctual. It breaks my heart to think he's retiring soon.

As I sit in his examining room, I feel terrible. Even though it's the middle of summer, I have my jacket wrapped around me. It has been two weeks since my surgery, and I think I should be feeling great by this time. After all, it was just a run-of-the-mill prostate removal. My doctor never keeps his patients waiting long, and a moment or two later he was in the room with me. Right off the bat, I was touched by his concern. When he asked me how I was doing, I told him that I didn't know why, after two weeks, I still felt so rotten.

He was incredulous. He went on to inform me that having your prostate removed was a major surgery and that I could expect to feel pretty low for a while. I told him I had no idea, and that was the truth, as almost *no patient education had taken place prior to my surgery.*

I've shared this story with family and friends and many felt that the fault lie with me for not going on-line and thoroughly researching what the surgery involved. Their thought was that I should have educated myself and then pressed the doctor for more information. One friend told me, "You have to be aggressive when it comes to questioning your doctor and getting all the necessary information." My response to this is BULLSHIT! I'm the patient. My job is to show up on time and get cured. How in God's name should I be the one responsible for educating myself about prostate surgery?

Tomorrow, I am taking my car in for a front end alignment. We are blessed to have a very good mechanic who can actually fix things. I promise you that I am not going to do on-line research about front end alignments before I go to see him. That's not my job; it's not my responsibility. My function is to show up with a broken car and leave with a repaired one.

But the human body isn't a car, is it? I don't need to have a heart-to-heart talk with my car before the alignment to explain what it is about to go through. There isn't a need to tell my car about post-alignment issues that may occur.

There was however the expectation that I, as the patient, would be told about how difficult this surgery was going to be and how long the recovery would take. A further expectation was that I would be educated about the after effects of surgery.

So let's do a little Q&A, shall we.
- Did you know that incontinence is a very common after-effect of a prostatectomy?
    - WELL NEITHER DID I!
- Did you know that a man's penis will be shorter after a prostatectomy?
    - WELL NEITHER DID I!
- Did you know impotence is a common after effect of a prostatectomy?
    - This one I actually did know, but not because my doctor told me.

- Did you know I would have an increased chance of a 'secondary' cancer following my prostatectomy?
  - WELL NEITHER DID I!

Christ, I get so angry when I think back on this. All of this could have been covered during any one of my pre-surgery visits, but it wasn't. Maybe my family and friends are right; maybe the fault lies with me for not researching everything about prostate removal. Maybe these people were right, but in my heart, I don't think they are. I absolutely believe it is the doctor's responsibility to take ownership of patient education. One of the problems with the patient taking responsibility for his own medical education is that he will most certainly do his research on-line, and on-line information can be all over the board.

Take prostate screening and testing as an example as discussed earlier in the book. (Please, feel free to go on-line and confuse the hell out of yourself). There is very little agreement in the medical community about:

- When a man should be tested
- If a man should be tested
- What the test should be
- How the results of the test should be interpreted

These seem like relatively simple questions, but apparently they are not, as there are no simple or agreed upon answers.

Let's research something simple. What is the answer to the question, "What percentage of men will struggle with incontinence following prostate surgery?" That seems like a fair question and also a question that approximately 150% of the men having a prostatectomy would want to know the answer to. Most medical websites don't even quantify an answer in percentage form as they, too, may be confused by what the right number is. When I did find a percentage posted, there was no consistency in the numbers reported. I found numbers that ranged between 1% to 98%. In other words, the results were meaningless. One of the more inane reasons for this confusion is that doctors can't even come to an agreement on what constitutes incontinence. If you can't agree on a definition; you can't successfully quantify it, can you?

So, we briefly relooked at PSA numbers and incontinence and realize there is confusion. Anybody out there still think I should be responsible for my own education?

I'm a writer and spend many hours doing research for my books. My fourth novel, *'A Prairie Fortnight'* was a novelization of the events surrounding the 1832 Indian Creek Massacre, which took place not all that far from where I live. Because this was a real event, involving real people, the need for accurate research was crucial. Oftentimes my research, instead of clarifying these historical events, confused them. There was a plethora of contradictory information to wade through in the hopes of finding the correct information. Was it frustrating? You bet it was.

The internet is a wonderful tool for so many reasons and for so many applications. I give it five-stars if I need to know the weather or traffic or to search a sale or a movie start time. When it comes to educating a layman on important medical questions, I would step cautiously.

Because of my radiation induced lymph issues, I was under the care of a physiatrist for a short period. I absolutely loved this Doctor, and even though I don't go to see her anymore, I still have great respect for her. Plus, I really liked her, which earns big points when I evaluate a medical professional. Shortly into my first appointment, she had a heart-to-heart with me about staying off the internet for medical advice. She made me promise her that if I had any questions, I would call her office and get my answers and advice from them. Because of what a physiatrist does, she didn't want patients trying things that might do more harm than good.

My physiatrist is not alone in her thinking about patients using the internet as a way to educate and, in many cases, diagnose and treat themselves. Dr. Google is available twenty-four hours a day, and you don't need insurance or an appointment to go see him. One issue is that patients who show up for an appointment with an armload of printouts from various websites will surely clog the system as doctors will need to spend more time with that patient. A second concern is the amount of data you will get back from a Google search. For example, I searched 'prostate surgery' and got, are you ready for this, 97,700,000 results. Most people, including me, will look at several of these sites before saying, "No mas", so there's no way to tell if you have reviewed the best information from your search.

We need to close the circle on my prostate removal. I went through the surgery and struggled through a long and painful recovery. A recovery I was unprepared for. Dear Reader, I will honestly share with you that I was impacted with every side effect that has been discussed in this chapter; side-effects that had never been discussed with me prior to surgery.

Perhaps the legitimate question might be, *"What difference would it have made if I knew all of this beforehand?"* Would it have made the surgery less intrusive? Would I have had a shorter recovery? Would it have been a less painful recovery? Would better patient education have meant that I might not have to deal with some of these chronic after-effects? The truth is that better patient education would not have moved the needle on any of those things, but that doesn't mean that it wouldn't have made a difference. The difference is I would have been better prepared for what to expect, and that in my book, would have made a huge difference.

I thought this quote from Dr. Cathy MacLean would be a good way to close this chapter. It is from an article she submitted in 2010. It is still as relevant today as it was ten-years ago. Thank you Dr. MacLean for granting me the permission to include this quote in the book, and thank you for your continued efforts to educate doctors on the importance of educating patients.

Sharing a Passion, Sharing Resources
By Cathy MacLean, MD MClSc MBA FCFP

The Latin word for doctor is docere, *which means* to teach. *To achieve shared decision making, improve understanding and adherence, motivate, and encourage self-management, **we have to be effective patient educators** and work well with other health providers who share this role.*

Chapter Twelve: Stupid things people say to people with cancer

The title of this chapter may surprise you unless you are a cancer patient, survivor, or a caregiver; then you probably know exactly what I'm talking about. Perhaps you might ask, *"Why would anyone say something stupid to a cancer patient?"* And my reply would be, "I don't know, they just do." Is there really a need for this chapter or is it just your author stirring up trouble by crying 'Wolf!' in a crowded movie theatre? That's a fair question, so please; take a moment and Google, *'stupid things people say to people with cancer'*, and you will get multiple hits for whole websites dedicated to these phenomena.

I consider myself pretty fortunate as my family and friends don't seem to be quite as stupid as some of the clods I read about on these websites, even though I have had both family and friends who should have stopped and thought before saying anything. I realize that one issue is that people just aren't sure what to say to someone with cancer. Part of that is cancer's fault, as cancer comes in so many varieties and some people are inclined to think that some of these varieties are not so bad. Let me repeat myself, once again; there is no such thing as a good cancer. If you think your friend is lucky to *'only have melanoma'*, and you are so convinced that he's lucky to *'only have melanoma'*, that you actually tell him how lucky he is to *'only have melanoma'*; then you are an idiot.

All cancers are bad; scary bad, keep you awake at night bad, gut wrenching bad, cry when no one is looking bad. ALL cancers! It would behoove you to remember that when speaking to a cancer patient.

First, a word about stupid, as it really should be defined before we jump into this. Stupid, like cancer, comes in an assortment of flavors.

- There is:
  o Funny Stupid
  o Insensitive Stupid
  o Naïve Stupid
  o Too Smart for your own Good Stupid
  o Staring at the Sun Stupid

CANCER BABBLE

- o   Darwin Award Winning Stupid

Let's start with a non-cancer related look at someone being stupid because there is stupid all around us in this world. I mentioned my wife, Marilyn, is a huge Cubs fan. We have the game on a lot in the summer. I'm not much of a sports fan anymore, but I am a Marilyn fan, so I'll sit and watch games with her. We watch on a 55" Ultra-Hi-Def TV, which is a long way from the TVs I grew up with. Those had small, Black & White screens. Protruding from the back of the set were two antennas and, in the hopes of getting a better picture, at the end of each antenna we would add a clump of aluminum foil. There were times my father would strategically place me or my sisters at key points around the room; convinced that this would improve reception. Patience, we haven't even gotten to the stupid part yet...or maybe we have?

Wrigley Field is the place to be in Chicago in the summertime and Cubs tickets sell for a lot of money. I can't imagine what seats right behind home plate go for. You would have to be rich to afford them, but apparently, you don't have to be smart. How so? Please, read on. On our 55" Ultra-Hi-Def TV, you can clearly see the people in the first rows behind home plate. The picture is so clear it's like they're right in your living room with you. Invariably, there is someone in one of these uber-expensive seats with a phone to his ear talking to someone out in TV land. The whole time, this person is waving frantically at whoever is on the other end of the phone. Stop waving; we see you. Everybody in the world can see you. I'm pretty sure your friend can see you, but just to make sure; you better stay on the phone for the second and third inning, and continue talking to him and waving like a madman, just in case your friend is a complete moron or is perhaps legally blind. This one is a toss-up as I'm not sure who is stupider; the guy at the game or the person he's talking to. Rich and stupid always make for a fun combination.

That example might best be filed under funny stupid. Funny stupid isn't the worst kind of stupid when communicating with a cancer patient.

Who knows, it may be so stupid that the cancer patient might get a good laugh out of it, and it's good to make a cancer patient laugh.

Recently, during my third battle with cancer, shortly after my second chemo cycle, my hair fell out. I ran a brush through my hair, stopped to clear the mass of hair that had come out, and repeated. The majority of this fallout all happened in one morning. I had a full head of hair, including a ponytail, when I woke up that day, and by mid-morning, I was pretty much bald. Don't ask me why, but as I lost more hair, I would just keep piling it up on some paper towels. It was an impressive pile by the time I was done with this bizarre ritual. I took a picture of it and sent it to a friend of ours. For the life of me, I have no explanation for why I did this. Our dear friend, who lives in the desert, and was perhaps suffering from some sun induced dementia, saw the picture and replied, "Was that from the chemo?" Marilyn and I had a tremendous laugh at that, so much so that we called our friends that night to thank them for the laugh. We laughed even harder when his wife said, "I told him that was a stupid thing to say." She was right, but there are times when stupid funny can be a very good thing.

When I found out that I would be losing my bladder during this third dance with the devil, I was understandably concerned. I had already lost my prostate, and was now going to lose my bladder, and couldn't help wondering how many body parts I could afford to lose before I should really start worrying. My doctor told me that people can live somewhat normal lives without a bladder. That's good to know. I took comfort when anyone would tell me about people they knew who were functioning without a bladder. A friend told me, via e-mail, that years ago his father's bladder, *"...blew up after eating a bad salad"*, and that his bladder had been removed and that his dad was doing fine. No, I'm not making that up. I was anxious to talk to my friend about how his father was functioning without a bladder, as well as to hear more about this sinister sounding salad. While on the phone, I came to the slow realization that his father had actually lost his *gallbladder* and that the man still had his bladder. My friend's comment was, "Isn't that the same thing?" Again, we laughed.

94

If it could all be funny stupid, I probably wouldn't be writing this chapter. But unfortunately, it is not. I mentioned earlier in the book that the American Cancer Society sponsors Relay for Life events, in part, as a celebration for cancer survivors. I have attended at least one Relay for Life every year for the past thirteen years, and each year, I have been given a purple 'survivor' tee-shirt that I wear with pride. One day, while in a store, the clerk looked at my shirt and said, "I was part of that event, but my tee-shirt was white. I would have rather had a purple one." She just didn't realize that the purple shirts were reserved for cancer patients-survivors. It was an innocent mistake. I sort of laughed and replied, "Believe me; you don't want a purple shirt. It means you had cancer." The following is an example of insensitive stupid. Her indignant reply was, "I may not have had cancer, but I have had plenty of other health issues."

On a related note, I mentioned that Abbey Road, our sort of a Black Lab, had cancer with me in 2018 and she has again joined me in cancer in 2019. Weird, huh? In 2018, we opted to have the tumor removed. We love her and just weren't ready to say goodbye to her yet. We are glad we did it as Abbey has had a wonderful quality of life since the surgery. She's thirteen now, and will most certainly break our hearts one day, but that day is not today. When I picked her up from the vet, she was wearing the 'cone-of-shame'. I was letting her air herself on the front lawn when a neighbor walked over. She expressed concern about the dog, which was very thoughtful. I told her that Abbey and I were both going through cancer at the same time at which point she said, "So, a lot of people have cancer." She seemed angry as she said it. Without another word, she turned and walked off. That brief encounter was over a year ago.

A year later, I still wonder at where the hostility came from, not just from my neighbor but also from the store clerk. Out of all the things both of these women could have said, they chose to say something stupid, hurtful, and insensitive. Why?

A college friend, who I had not spoken to for more than a few years, found out that I had cancer and gave me a call. His agenda in calling was to tell me that as we get older, we all have to deal with health issues and that if I thought I was going to get any sympathy from him, then I, and I quote, "...had come to the wrong place."

Wait, what?

I mentioned (at length) that I was unprepared for how difficult my prostate removal (prostatectomy) would be, not only to get through it but also to recover from. Many weeks after the surgery, I was still laid pretty low. I felt bad, and I sure didn't feel any better when I received a phone call from a family member who told me repeatedly that having a prostate removed was no big deal. "It's nothing," she said. Evidently, she knew numerous men who had their prostates removed, and I was the only wimpy, candy-ass who struggled with it. That one left a mark.

We became reacquainted with an old friend, who we hadn't seen in years. She was fundraising for a breast cancer event she was involved in. Even though I am not big on social media, I saw on-line that she had posted a lot about breast cancer. She reached out to me to thank me for the donation. I mentioned that I had cancer and hesitantly asked her if she was a breast cancer survivor. She informed me that 'no', she hadn't had cancer, but she had *almost had cancer*, not once but several times. To this day I have no idea what that meant. She never did ask me about my cancer but shared with me at length the horrors of *almost* having cancer. I wanted to ask her what was worse; *almost* having chemo or *almost* having radiation. Thank God she didn't have to go through the anguish of *almost* having surgery.

Beware of the positivity police. They are definitely naïve stupid with strong leanings towards insensitive stupid. They are convinced that the key to your recovery has to do with having a positive attitude. I believe having a good attitude is more beneficial than having a negative attitude, and I believe I'm a pretty typical cancer patient when I tell you that I do try to keep the negative thoughts at bay. Recently we were out with friends when my friend's wife decided that I needed to be convinced of just how important a positive attitude is. She fixed me with an intense stare, and said, "You know, you have to have a positive attitude." I agreed with her, but evidently I was not very convincing as she opted to repeat just how important attitude is. I agreed again. This time I really did try to look positive; I was grinning like an idiot in the hopes of showing her just how positive I was. I'm sure I looked deranged. Still not convinced, she launched into another diatribe about the importance of positivity. OK, three times is two times too many to listen to that crap. I'm not proud of this, but I told her my positivity quotient was fine on most days, and when she has had cancer for the third time; she should look me up and then we can have a meaningful talk about attitude. Sadly, at the end of the day, all I accomplished was to convince her that I really had a lousy attitude and really needed to be more positive. Looking back on it, I guess that makes me stupid, too.

An old friend from out of town was visiting, and another friend hosted a small get together at her home. We both love these little reunions and seeing our old friends. They knew I was going through cancer treatments at the time. They were used to seeing me with a full head of hair so my chrome-dome was a bit shocking. Our hostess grabbed her computer and started showing pictures of a family member who had died from cancer. He looked healthy and robust at first, but this poor man, who, by the way, I didn't know personally, looked worse and worse in each picture. By the time she got to the last pictures, he was little more than a skeleton. I don't know why anyone would have taken these pictures in the first place, and I certainly couldn't understand why someone would show them to a cancer patient (at a party of all places). You, Dear Reader, didn't see these pictures, but trust me when I say they were haunting, and that I'll never get some of those images out of my head.

Marilyn's mother died years ago from ovarian cancer. Needless to say, it was a difficult time for the entire family. My wife told her best friend, whose mother incidentally had also passed from cancer, about her mom's cancer. The friend could only repeat (and repeat, and repeat), "How did this happen? I don't understand how this could happen. Cancer? How did she get cancer?" Twenty-five years later and these comments still nag at my wife.

Stupid questions are high on the list of stupid things people say to people with cancer.

- Please don't ask:
    - How could this happen?
    - Have you seen a doctor?
    - Are you sure it's cancer?
    - Did you smoke?
    - What kind of odds are they giving you?
    - Do you have life insurance?
    - What stage are you?
    - Did you use talcum powder?
    - Did you get a second opinion?
    - Can you sue someone? (I threw that in because of all the ads I see on TV)
    - Are you kidding?

I was still in my twenties when my dad passed away. There was no surprise as he was in his eighties and had suffered from bad health, including cancer, for several years before he passed. None of that made losing him any easier. On the day he died, I went to my folk's house and cut their grass. I was feeling lost and didn't know what else to do, so why not do that? The entire time I was engaged in this mindless task, I fought back tears. His neighbor approached me, and I told him my father was gone. He said, "You're kidding, right?" No, I assured him, my father had passed. "You got to be kidding me," he said again. This peculiar ritual went back and forth several more times like a really bad Abbott and Costello routine. I didn't know what he wanted me to say, and all I wanted was for him to SHUT UP and quit repeating the same stupid and insensitive things. This conversation took place in 1981. If I'm telling you about this encounter 38-years later, you can be pretty sure that it left a scar.

Here's an important safety tip for you. If someone tells you they have cancer, please don't ask them if they are kidding unless you delight in coming across as a complete ass-hat.

When I decided to include this as a chapter, I committed to only include stories that involved me or people I know, even though, as I mentioned, you could spend all day reading web sites dedicated to this subject. I reached out to friends who had dealt with cancer and asked if they might be willing to share their stories.

This first one is from a friend of mine, a nurse, who went through breast cancer about the same time I was going through my first cancer (circa 2007). I learned a lot about breast cancer from her, and the lesson I came away with is that breast cancer treatment goes on for a really long time. It's exhausting for the patient. My friend went through chemo, and radiation, and finally multiple surgeries. I respect anyone who goes through cancer, but that goes double for those with breast cancer or any cancer where the patient's treatments get dragged out over many months.

She sent me the following, and at first, I looked at how I might edit it. I read it several times and realized that I didn't want to change a word. If I was to create a category for this it would be: *even really smart, educated people* (in this case a doctor and radiation technicians) *can be really stupid.*

Most of the cancer care that I received was good, and some of the care was quite excellent. I had only one really awful experience. It occurred during my radiation treatments.

The treatment required that I have both my arms raised up over my head in order to maximize the area of my chest that was being radiated. The first few treatments were uneventful.

Unfortunately, at about the time of my fourth or fifth treatment, I was doing something at home and injured my right shoulder. It was

99

extremely painful for me to raise my arm up in order to fit in my body mold. (Author's Note: you are 'mapped' for radiation and a mold is made. This ensures you are in the same position for each treatment)

A couple of times I asked the radiation tech if there was a different way to position me, or if there was anything else we could do. I was told that I needed to discuss it with the doctor the next time I saw her. I totally understood and agreed with that answer since I knew that the techs were not qualified to make that determination.

My next appointment with the doctor was more than a week away. I didn't particularly want to experience that extreme shoulder pain every day, so I asked to move my appointment to a sooner date. I was told that she was totally booked and there was nothing available any sooner. I was told that if the pain was unbearable that I could always go to the emergency room.

Of course, I did not go to the ER. I just went to my daily treatments and tried to get through it as best I could. All things considered, I thought I did well. However, the radiation techs must have had a different opinion.

When the date of my appointment finally arrived, my doctor immediately told me that she was informed that I was "having problems". What was portrayed to her was that I said that the positioning and the treatments were the cause of my pain. She never gave me a chance to explain anything different. She then went on to say that she had treated hundreds of women just like me, and none of them have pain, so what's my problem?

Needless to say, I was shocked. The only response I could come up with was, "Are you kidding?"

When I recovered, I said that we should follow her logic a little further. I told her that I knew hundreds of women, who all have breasts, and none of them have cancer, so does that mean that I don't have it either?

After that exchange, she and I just tolerated each other, which made my remaining 30+ treatments dreadful.

That story really pisses me off. It is not only a case of smart people being stupid; it is an excellent example of the insensitivity on the part of some in the health care profession. To recap, this doctor has a cancer patient who is in pain and yet she can't clear a few minutes of her schedule to see her. You, doctor, should leave the medical profession IMMEDIATELY! I'd like to punch her doctor in the throat. My friend's husband is a black belt, and I know he can hit a lot harder than I can, so I hope he decides to throw that well deserved punch instead.

At about the time I was starting my third bout with cancer, I found out an old friend had been diagnosed with stage IV liver cancer. We have grown close during these last few months, and I'm glad he's been part of my life this summer. When I mentioned *CANCER BABBLE*, and my 'stupid things people say' chapter, he shared the following hurtful stupid comment.

When he told his friend about the cancer, the friend's comment was, "Isn't that what Walter Peyton died from?"

This may be a good moment to segue into a few ground rules that we should all follow when talking to a cancer patient:

- Rule 1: My cancer is my cancer. It is not your neighbor's, brother's, coworker's, uncle's cancer so please don't share some third party information about some guy I don't know.
- Rule 2: If your neighbor's, brother's, coworker's, uncle died from his cancer, please don't feel compelled to share that information with me.

The same friend from above, with the stage IV liver cancer, bought a second life insurance policy years before his diagnosis. A friend of his knew of this purchase, and when my friend was diagnosed, his friend told him, "I'll bet you're glad now that you bought that second insurance policy."

The following is from a friend who survived breast cancer. I'd categorize this comment as Award Winning Stupid.

From my friend: *I was talking to a woman whom I thought was intelligent and would be able to distinguish between things that are good and pleasurable as opposed to things that are bad & uncomfortable. Therefore, I never expected to hear her say something so clearly ridiculous. Perhaps I should cut her a little slack because she's never had cancer so obviously she never needed treatment...but still...*

Anyway, this woman was asking me how far along I was with my treatments. I told her that I had completed three chemo sessions & had five more to go.

She replied that I must really look forward to my chemo days because the chemo clinic is "like a day at the spa". She explained to me that chemo patients relax in big comfy reclining chairs. And for several hours they just chill out, watch TV, read a book, or take a nap.

"Sounds like heaven to me."

Another friend, who coincidently was also going through breast cancer treatment at about the same time as my first cancer, was good enough to share some of her experiences with me. She was an industry friend of mine, but we didn't work in the same office or even in the same part of the business, but we would still run into each other occasionally. I like to think that those were special days for both of us, not just because we shared a cancer background, but because we just seemed to have a nice connection between us. That, and she was funny and I'm happy to say that cancer did little to diminish her sense of humor. In truth, it was just the opposite. I asked her one day about post-treatment follow up screening.

From my friend, *"...the radiation oncologist who checked me out after the last treatment, and saw no burns or issues, recommended I come see her every three months for I don't know how long. To look at nothing wrong and do nothing about nothing wrong. Obviously she needed a kitchen remodel? I never went back."*

Evidently her radiation oncologist and medical oncologist went to the same medical school, because her experiences with both were similar.

From my friend, *"...So, chemo and radiation are over, and the oncologist also wants to see me every three months. The appointment* consisted of waiting in the Reception Area for 45 minutes past my appointment time, then sitting in that little cold room with nothing to do while waiting for the doctor for another ½ hour. The doctor finally comes in, and asks "How are you feeling?" I say, "Fine." He checks the boob out, and says, "Great, I'll see you in three months." During all that time he never ordered any sort of test or scans or anything. Just a 'great, see you in three months.'

She quit going back to see this guy as well.

The medical community has a name for cancer survivors: Renewable Resource. It's typical for doctors to conduct follow ups, and I'm not going to argue with the wisdom of that, but in my friend's case, she would tell me that they weren't doing anything. "A quick squeeze of the boob and come see me again in three months." She was my friend, and I wanted her to have the proper follow-up care, but instead, she got disillusioned and just quit going and that's not good either. So, does what happened to her qualify as stupid? Yes, I believe it does, and if I had to categorize it, I might call it scary stupid.

I had a similar experience with follow-up after my 2007 bout with anal cancer. My oncologist kept sending me for CT scans every couple of months. My primary doctor was copied on the results of these scans, and I'm happy to say the scan results were good. During my next visit with my primary doctor, he asked me why I was going for so many CT scans. My less than brilliant response was, "Because they tell me to." His concern was that I had had a belly-full of radiation already and CT scans added to that total. CT scans can expose you to as much radiation as 200 chest X-rays. As a patient, that put me in a tough spot as I liked and respected both of these doctors, and whether or not I needed these scans was absolutely not my call. A patient always wants to operate from the point of view that, no matter what test you are being sent for, that test is vital to your well-being.

Much of what you can and can't say to a cancer patient depends on what type of relationship you have with the person. If you have always had an open and frank relationship, then you can probably get away with being open and frank in your discussion about cancer. I have had a friend for years, and it is rare for me to be with this person where we aren't hurling insults at one another. We love each other. The insults are just the way we communicate. I'm not sure why this is; it just is. For his sake, I sometimes wish it was different as he's not good at sarcasm and cynicism. For me, when I get into one of these battles of wits with him, it's like fighting an unarmed man.

If he ever approached me all mealy-mouthed and sad over my cancer, I know that would make me feel just awful. If he comes at me with barbs and insults, then I have to believe that I'm going to be OK. If someone was to witness one of our exchanges, they would probably be shocked. They would probably consider my friend a horrible person for talking to a cancer patient like that. They would be right about that most of the time, but not in this case. Please keep in mind that this banter is only acceptable under these very special circumstances.

There have been a few times that people tried to 'bring the funny' when they approached me about cancer. It didn't work because that was not the nature of our relationship. I think their hearts were in the right place, but they really should have thought of a different approach.

Another important safety tip that you should understand is that the cancer patient is being bombarded by some pretty potent drugs. There are days during treatment when they might be feeling physically and emotionally good, and on other days; not so much. The problem is you can't tell by looking at them where they are at along this emotional spectrum. My current chemo-cocktail is a combination of Carboplatin and Etoposide, and I am happy to report that I have had very few adverse effects from these drugs. But just because I have not had to deal with nausea, diarrhea, vomiting, mouth sores, etc. don't think these drugs aren't in the background doing all their nasty chemo stuff. Weekly, I go for 'labs' which determines how my blood is dealing with the chemo. The answer, as I prepare for my fourth chemo cycle, is not too good. In other words, my immune system is getting the crap beat out of it. I'm under house arrest, or at least that's how it feels. No handshakes, no hugs, no kisses, no malls, no restaurants, no church, no theaters; well, I guess you get the idea. I'm tired a lot and this fatigue definitely impacts me emotionally. So yes, I am back to crying when I see commercials for St. Jude's Children's Hospital or those commercials about abused animals. On days that I'm doing better emotionally, you can probably get away with saying something stupid to me and I might not react or even notice. When I'm experiencing a down-tic, those same comments will affect me much more.

I hope you liked this chapter; it went on for longer than I thought it would. Sadly, a chapter about stupid things people say to cancer patients will end up being the longest chapter in the book. In truth, I could have made it a lot longer. Is there a lesson hidden in there somewhere? If nothing else, I believe it shows that it was necessary to include this as a topic.

Let's see if we can sum it up. Because you can't be sure where a cancer patient is physically and emotionally on any given day, my advice to you is to tread softly. Think before you speak. Start out with a verbal hug or perhaps a real hug if the right words just won't seem to come. You may be glad you did, as there are days when a cancer patient is going to have less tolerance for stupid things you might say. Besides, there is always a chance that the cancer patient may write a book one day, and in that book he may include a chapter entitled, *Stupid things people say to people with cancer*, and you wouldn't want to be included in that chapter. Right?

Chapter Thirteen: The Zen of writing and how it relates to cancer

I was awake in the middle of the night again last night. This wasn't related to any drug that I was taking; sometimes I just wake up and end up staying awake for a while. I mentioned earlier that as a writer, this isn't necessarily a bad thing as it gives me quiet time to think about the next day's writing. Most writers mentally write much of a book when they are nowhere near their laptop or writing pad. Waking up during the night bothers me even less now that I'm retired. When I was still working, and getting up at 4:45am every morning, these middle of the night awakenings could be very stressful.

Writing is more than my hobby. It has become my passion over the past seven-years. I love writing, but I do almost nothing to promote myself as a writer or to market my books. I did however motivate myself to attend a seminar one day on successful marketing and was told that I would need to dedicate 40% of my time to promoting my books. That would be 40% of my time that I'm not writing, and I wasn't willing to make that tradeoff. I work in anonymity, and I'm fine with that. I believe that my writing will one day receive some level of notoriety, but I won't be the catalyst for that happening. I may not even notice; I'll be too busy writing.

In 2013, when I sat down to write my first novel, *CLEARING*, I realized pretty quickly that I needed to have a game plan if I hoped to complete this task. Fortunately for me, I've always been task oriented. As an example, in the past, when working on my stained glass, I would commit to working on a project every day with no exceptions. All too often, I would see other people who would put aside their project for one day; just one day, but invariably, one day would become two, and two would become four, and at some point the project would be abandoned. Have you ever been in someone's home and discovered a downstairs bathroom that was partially demolished, two years earlier, in preparation for remodeling, and nothing had been done to it since to complete the project. See, that was a guy who didn't have the discipline going into it. He lacked vision. He needed a game-plan, and all good game-plans need three things; a beginning, a middle, and an end.

Stained glass projects have a complexity to them that goes well beyond creating a pattern and choosing colors. I know going into it that I may need twenty or twenty-five separate sessions to bring the work to fruition. First, I need to cut, grind, and fit the glass pieces. Following that, the pieces need to be cleaned and foiled before they are soldered together. Another session or two is needed to clean the solder and patina the lead. The same is true for the U-shaped zinc channel for the outside border of the piece. Penultimately, there's milling the sections for the wood frame. This includes staining and varnishing the pieces. Finally, comes the hardware and installation.

Before I touched a stained glass project, I would visualize what it would take to get from the beginning of the project to the end. There were times that I would come up with a pattern that I liked, and then say, forget it. I worried whether I would have the time or the discipline to complete it. The key word in that last statement is 'discipline'. I was blessed to have the discipline to stick with the projects that I started, but there were always going to be days that I had zero interest in working on my glass. On those days, I would make a deal with myself to cut one-piece of glass. Just one and that would fulfill my obligation. Invariably, once I sat down at my work bench, I would get lost in the work and cut more than just the one piece. Some of those low motivation days would blossom into some of my most productive sessions.

Creating a stained glass window takes time, commitment, and discipline but it is still nowhere near to what it takes to write a book. When I sit down to write a book, I know that as much as one year could go by before that book is on the shelf; and that's now that I'm retired. When I was still working, my first two books took closer to eighteen months to complete. If building a stained glass window is a 5K run, then writing a book is a triathlon. I've done library talks in the past on the discipline of writing and how to create production goals for yourself as a writer. I discuss how to make a game plan that ensures you will be successful. At some point during these talks I dust off the old joke, "How do you eat an elephant?"

The answer, of course, is, 'One bite at a time'.

Thank you, Dear Reader, for indulging me for a few moments. I really do have a point in leading you down this path. Cancer patients, just like stained glass artists and writers, need commitment. The cure takes time; in some cases a lot of time. You need a game plan to get through cancer, and as I mentioned earlier, all good game-plans need three things; a beginning, middle, and an end. Cancer can be exhausting, but you can't give up on it. During this third go-around with cancer, I'm getting a real feel for just how exhausting it really is. It will equate to a year out of my life to get through this, and that's under the proviso that things work out OK. A year is best case scenario. A year of being poked and prodded; a year of lab work and doctor's appointments; a year that will include multiple days of sitting in chemoland as poison is pumped into me; a year of scans; a year of anxiously awaiting the results of those scans. And at some point, there will be surgery and waking up minus a bladder, and the transition to living without an organ that has been with me for sixty-six years. I have to understand all of this before I ever venture down this path. I need to see and understand the intricate landscape that has been laid out before me. I need to understand where the beginning is, and what it will take to get through the middle, and ultimately, how it will all end.

I'm not a strong person, but I don't have the luxury of being weak.

I am not tough, but will have to galvanize my resolve for this battle.

This journey is not for the timid, but I question where the courage will come from to navigate myself through this.

Cancer is an elephant, and I ask myself, 'How do you eat an elephant?'

Well, you know.

As of today, August 19, 2019, I am 37,000 words into *CANCER BABBLE*. While I lie awake during the night I am struck with a bizarre thought. This may surprise you, but like a lot of writers, I do not work from an outline. As I write, I have a vague idea where the story is headed and, at some point, I will have a pretty good idea of how the story will end. In my first four books, by this point, I had a good feel for how the story would resolve itself. That's not the case with CANCER BABBLE, as I'm not writing the end.

The end is being written for me.

Have you ever thrown a piece of driftwood into a fast moving creek and watch as the wood bobs along and caroms off rocks and branches? I have as much control over the last chapter of this book as that piece of driftwood has over its own fate.

Try to get that thought out of your head and go back to sleep as you lie awake in the quiet darkness of two o'clock in the morning.

Chapter Fourteen: Chemo-Brain

Chemo-brain; hold on a minute; what were we talking about? Oh yeah, chemo-brain. Wait, I forgot what I was going to say about chemo-brain. Well, now you get the point. Chemo-brain is a side effect of chemotherapy. It can also be called chemo fog or if you prefer fancier labels; cancer-related cognitive impairment or cognitive dysfunction. In laymen's terms, you can get totally zoned out on that chemo shit, man.

Like everything else on the internet, you will find conflicting information about chemo-brain. Not everyone agrees on what it is or what causes it. There are some in the medical community who believe that, like Bigfoot, UFOs, and Episcopalians, it does not really exist.

The following list of symptoms related to chemo-brain is from the Mayo Clinic website

- Being unusually disorganized
- Confusion
- Difficulty concentrating
- Difficulty finding the right word
- Difficulty learning new skills
- Difficulty multitasking
- Feeling of mental fogginess
- Short attention span
- Short-term memory problems
- Taking longer than usual to complete routine tasks
- Trouble with verbal memory, such as remembering a conversation
- Trouble with visual memory, such as recalling an image or list of words

I am understandably concerned after reviewing this list as I was evidently born with chemo-brain and have been a victim of it my entire life. All of these things, to a certain extent, apply to me, and as much as I would like to blame my 'air-headedness' on chemo, I can't in good faith do that. I'm pretty sure I would have remembered getting chemotherapy in grade school, but I know I didn't, and yet, I was one of the bigger space-cadets in grammar school and high school. Even back then, I was checking off every one of the boxes on that list.

I am a baby boomer who grew up in Chicago in the fifties and sixties. Our post WW-II parents were procreating like there was no tomorrow and the result was that we had kids coming out of the woodwork. Neighborhoods, and therefore schools, were overcrowded. My grade school had over forty kids to a classroom with one teacher. There were no helpers or teacher's aides in the classroom, just one overworked, stressed-out, and often borderline psychotic teacher. The cognitive level within this overcrowded Petrie dish of a classroom ranged from genius IQ to functionally retarded, and please don't get all PC on me. Retarded was an acceptable way of describing certain kids during that period. One of my best friends in grade school was retarded. He was one of the few kids I looked smart standing next to. From that point of view, I was glad to have him in class with me.

And where did I, your humble author, fall within this grey-matter spectrum? That's a good question. I never considered myself to be stupid, and yet I did lousy in school, and trust me; I brought home the horrible report cards to validate this. I never heard the term Attention Deficit Disorder (ADD) while growing up. Years later, I realized that I was a textbook example of someone with ADD. There were days, in truth most days, in which I had completely checked-out five minutes into the school day, and that was it; game over as nothing was going to seep in for the rest of the day. I thought that this was perfectly normal. I thought I was ordinary and that all the other kids stood shoulder to shoulder with me as I drifted through the hazy fog of each new day.

So here I sit decades later and still battle Attention Deficit Disorder on a daily basis. I had a boss who I liked a great deal, but he was long winded. It took him a long time to get to the point. I was comfortable enough in my relationship with him to remind him that I had ADD and that it was in his best interest to communicate with me using twenty-five words or less. Here's an important safety tip for those of you who need to deal with someone with ADD: Keep it short, simple, and to the point.

So now I find out that scooped over the top of my ADD, like thick gravy, is a smothering ladleful of chemo-brain. Please keep in mind that this may be the chemo-brain talking, but I don't remember chemo-brain being discussed in 2007 when I went through my first round of cancer. I knew at the time that I had ADD, but I think I would have remembered something as impacting as chemo-brain. For instance, if a doctor had told me, "We are about to start your chemotherapy, and you are about to get a whole lot stupider." I think I would have a vivid recollection of that conversation.

Looking back on it, now that I finally found out about this whole chemo-brain thing, I did see evidence of it. When I went back to work in 2007 after that first bout with cancer, I had to stop and think of people's names. I'm talking about people that I knew well and had worked with for years. My guess is that a lot of people might have been concerned about these mental lapses but, in truth, I hardly gave it a second thought. Maybe when you live with ADD for your whole life you just accept these cognitive dropouts as normal. That's kind of weird, right?

When you are prescribed chemotherapy for the treatment of cancer, you will be asked to attend a 'chemo-class'. That's a real thing. I'm not making that up. The class Marilyn and I attended in 2007 was a farce. While Marilyn and I were hoping to gain some deeper insight into this strange new cancer world, the instructor's agenda was to get rid of us as quickly as possible. There was no mention of chemo-brain at that time but that was either because it wasn't recognized as a side effect in 2007 or perhaps because it was such a poorly conducted class that it just never came up. The chemo-class I went through in the spring of 2019 was a much better experience as it actually taught me something. The instructor took it seriously and that's what made the difference. It was during this recent class that I heard the term 'chemo-brain' for the first time.

Given the fact that I am not the brightest guy in the world, coupled with the news that my cognitive ability may be affected by my chemo drugs...well, let's just say that kind of information tends to get your attention. I immediately begin to look for evidence of chemo-brain. Our favorite television show is Jeopardy. Marilyn and I have recorded this show every afternoon for many years and watch it together every night. Jeopardy is a feast or famine kind of show as some nights we come away feeling pretty smart. Other nights, well let's just say there are some nights we don't feel quite so bright. The thing with trivia is that it's only hard if you don't know the answer, and some nights, we know fewer answers. As we both understand this to be a truth, we don't get too knotted up over it. C'est la vie, right? Even on those less than stellar nights, we still enjoy the challenge and feel we have learned something. Now that I know about chemo-brain, I need to worry about whether I'm just having a bad night at Jeopardy or if there is something more sinister at work here. One thing I can honestly tell you is that recently when watching Jeopardy, there are a lot of answers that I know I know, but I can't get the answer out. Picture it like this, the answer is stuck in my brain like a vending machine candy bar that has been bought and paid for but refuses to take the leap.

The toughest non-Jeopardy related question I now need to answer is, "Am I getting stupider?"

And of course you can't ask yourself that question without also asking the follow up question, "If I am getting stupider, exactly how much stupider can I expect to get?"

I think I'm OK getting a little dumber as no one has been asking me to explain quantum physics to them recently. Full disclosure here, no one has ever asked me to explain quantum physics to them, and thank God for that, as I'd be totally clueless. Quantum physics, please, I've never even fully understood how a toaster works.

But what if I don't just get a little dumber? What if I'm on my way to drooling into a rag and not knowing my own name? Well, there's a pretty fair chance I'm already heading to that point even without the chemo drugs in my diet, but I don't want to do anything to accelerate the process.

Crap, I wish I had never heard of chemo-brain.

We all have what's known as, 'Senior Moments'. By way of explanation, it is those times where the synapses in the brain just aren't firing correctly and you might end up doing something inexplicable. Have you ever looked for your glasses only to discover that you are wearing them? That's a senior moment. You go into the kitchen to get something, but once you're in there, you can't remember what you needed. Yep, that's another senior moment. You're driving and look down to see that your turn signal is on, and you have no idea how long it's been blinking away. You lose your train of thought mid-sentence. You can't remember the name of the book you just finished, and where the hell are my goddamn keys! It's sort of fun listing these things, and I could keep going, but you get the idea. Just so you know, I have been guilty of all of these mental lapses and plenty of others, too. When I was a young man, it was easier to just laugh off these little cognitive foibles. Now that I'm in my mid-sixties, they are more concerning. Let me qualify that a bit further; now that I'm in my mid-sixties, and have ADD, and also have chemo-brain to worry about, it becomes very concerning.

The answer to the question, "How concerned should I be?" becomes very subjective. If the worst thing that happens is not being able to spit out an answer on Jeopardy or misplacing my glasses, then I'm not too concerned at all. But what if that's not the worst of it? What if I forget to turn off the stove or if I leave the keys to the house dangling in the front door lock all night, or God forbid, I forget to put the toilet seat down?

Just as I do for almost everything, I conduct research on-line for the best information to share with you, Dear Reader, and I'm not making this up. I found this statement on one site in answer to the question, "How long does chemo-brain last?" Their answer: *For most patients, chemo-brain improves within 9-12 months after completing chemotherapy, but many people still have symptoms at the six-month mark.* I reread that line multiple times and even asked Marilyn to read it. We agreed it was worded oddly. I think whoever wrote that statement has chemo-brain, but at least I got a laugh out of it. It was akin to the sale papers when you read, "Save up to 40% ...or more."

CANCER BABBLE

I have had two agendas over the past several months; one is to talk to you about cancer and the other is to write a book. These goals, naturally, are related. When I write a book, at some point, I lose all objectivity. I don't know how it is for other authors, but after I get to around the thirty or forty thousand word mark, it is difficult for me to step far enough back from the work to honestly judge it. By comparison, I also do watercolor paintings. Notice I didn't say I'm a watercolor artist as that might mislead you into thinking I have some modicum of talent. When I complete a watercolor, I can look at my painting and easily and quickly assess whether or not I think it's any good.

This morning, I am approaching the forty-thousand word mark in *CANCER BABBLE,* and as I sit here at the word processor, I have to ask myself the toughest question of all, *"Is the book any good?"* Even more concerning is the question, *"Does it even make sense?"* Writers will probably understand what I'm saying, but I'm not sure if you, Dear Reader, will get my point.

I have had these moments of self-doubt on each of my first four books, but with *CANCER BABBLE* it is much more pronounced as I'm not telling a traditional story. In *CLEARING,* my first novel my main character, Billy, pretty much did exactly what I told him to do, when I told him to do it. Most of my characters from these first four books were well-behaved with the exception of a few characters that continually spit the bit and thundered off in a direction of their own choosing. (Usually for the betterment of the final product) As an aside, when a writer creates a character, they initially do all the talking and all the thinking for that character. At some point, our characters start to become more three-dimensional. They take on a life of their own and will gain a certain independence. This probably sounds insane, but when this happens, it is a wonderful moment for the writer and his 'children'. Yep, just reread that and it does sound crazy, but that doesn't make it any less true.

Assessing *CANCER BABBLE* is much more difficult than evaluating the other books. I have several wonderful people in my life who have been willing to read my books at various stages of completion and offer feedback.

This feedback has been invaluable, but I know I can't give them *CANCER BABBLE* in its current state and ask for them to review it.

I can tell you certain things about this latest book. I am in the later stages of this project. I can also tell you that, from my vantage point, my hunch is that it's a mess. I know I will have a lot of editing and rewrites at the end of the first draft as that is business as usual for any writer, but I can't honestly imagine what *CANCER BABBLE* will look like in its final incarnation.

I'm blaming the mess I'm in on two things. One is the nature of the book, as this book doesn't behave like a normal book. The second culprit that is conspiring to derail this project is chemo-brain. I told you I was looking for concrete evidence that chemo-brain is a real thing. Well, as of this morning, I may have a forty-thousand word example that proves the existence of chemo-brain.

Interlude Five: While I Pondered, Weak and Weary

August 23, 2019: I realized last night as I lie awake in the quiet, semi-darkness of my room that I have not given you an update in a while and there are several things I'd like to share with you. I did finally 'man-up' and contact the cemetery where my parents are buried. I asked, through their website, how one goes about purchasing two burial plots as I have no idea. I'm curious to know what it will cost. Am I tempting fate by reaching out to the cemetery? Maybe fate will work in my favor. You know, like when you lug an umbrella around with you all day, you can be pretty sure it won't rain. And let's say I do pull the trigger and purchase the plots. What's the worst that can happen; that I have them but won't need them at this time? There's not much of a downside as I know I'm going to use them eventually.

When they get back to me, I'll need to be prepared to answer questions that I've given little thought to during my lifetime. For instance, I'm not even sure if I'd prefer cremation or if I want to be embalmed. I'm a Catholic, albeit not a very good one, and the Catholic Church has wind-socked back and forth over the centuries with their stance concerning cremation. As of this writing, the Vatican gives cremation two thumbs up.

Weighing into my decision is this; there are so many zombie apocalypse books and movies out right now that I think cremation may be the prudent choice. I don't really believe that I will come back as a flesh craving abomination, but do I really want to take that chance?

This is the kind of crap I think of in the middle of the night. It's 2:00am and I'm awake, and it's dark, and I'm trying to chase these thoughts away, but they seem determined to plague me. They are rapping upon my chamber door with the persistence of Poe's accursed 'Raven'.

During my first two go-arounds with cancer, I never gave much thought to death. In 2007, my oncologist told me right off the bat that I had nothing to worry about and that this cancer was not going to kill me. God bless him, as that's what every cancer patient wants to hear. When cancer reappeared in my prostate, I foolishly considered that type of cancer as no big deal. Even though people die every day from prostate cancer, that thought never even entered my feeble little brain.

This time around, I am waiting for my oncologist and surgeon to assure me that I am going to be fine, but neither has said those magic words.

This is no time to be coy, people.

I need you to tell me this is just a bump in the road, and I'm going to be OK, and I need you to say it with conviction; like it's the most obvious thing in the world, and then laugh and ask me how could I possibly be this worried over something so inconsequential?

Is that asking too much?

But they haven't said it, and that does concern me.

Do you remember way back at the beginning of this book, when I told you that if you catch me in any moments of self-pity or self-wallowing you have my permission to toilet paper the trees in front of my house? You may want to swing by Wal-Mart and pick up a couple of rolls and head on over.

It is getting to be late August, and even though it is hard to believe, I'm staring Labor Day straight in the face. We are only given so many summers in our lifetime and this one is slipping away quickly. If I was still in school, and asked to write a composition entitled, "What I did on my summer vacation?" it would be a tragically short and uninteresting bit of writing. While others went on vacation; I went to chemoland, which is not nearly as much fun as Disneyland even though the lines are a lot shorter.

I watch the heavens perform their annual celestial magic as summer surrenders itself to the fall.

I know what this means as I've been to this rodeo many times.

The days are getting shorter; my life is getting shorter.

Chapter Fifteen: So what have I learned?

In a perfect world, we'd never stop learning. That seems to be a truth that most would agree with. Several chapters ago, I went on a rant about doctors who do a lousy job of educating their patients. Surfing the internet, I came away with the sense that these failures, on the part of many in the medical field, are chronic. Can I change the behavior of these doctors? It doesn't seem likely, and if I could, the best case is that I might influence one or two doctors, while so many others would plod along in their 'uneducating' way.

So, if I can't change the behavior of tens of thousands of doctors, the next best option is to change my own behavior. I met with my urologist/oncologist/surgeon (all the same guy) recently to discuss the removal of my bladder. I went in this time with the expectation that he would educate me on nothing prior to my surgery. That being the case, I spent a lot of time researching my upcoming procedure on my own. I am adamant when I say; I should not have had to do this. I'm the 'Cable-Guy'. If you want someone who can design a next generation, 1.2GHz, mid-split, fiber deep, dense-wave multiplexed system, come see me. If, on the other hand, you want to discuss the intricacies of getting your tonsils removed, keep walking as I can't help you with that, but perhaps you can help yourself.

Regardless of my personal opinions on who should teach whom, and when they should be taught, the reality seems to be that if you want to know what an upcoming medical procedure will be like, you had better be prepared to do your own homework. So that's exactly what I did. Bladder removal, as I was about to discover, comes in three flavors, so I focused my attention on the pros and cons of each of these approaches. For no particular reason, and in no particular order, I've listed the three options below, but I'll spare you the plusses and minuses or the details of each with exception of the one I chose. (Stay tuned for the exciting announcement!)

- Ileal Conduit (Urostomy)
- Continent Cutaneous Reservoir
- Orthotopic NeoBladder

I found images on-line for each of these options, which I printed and brought with me to the appointment. In addition, I put together a list of twenty-five bullet points related to the following five areas of concern.

- Which of the three surgical options makes the most sense for me?
- How is each surgery performed?
  - Open-Minimally Invasive-Robotic
- Which has the least chance of post-surgical issues?
  - Infections-Leakage-Blood Clots- Stones-Hernias-Lymph
- My goals
- Future concerns

I actually walked in with an opinion on which way I wanted to go when it came to the three surgical options that were available. In my layman's opinion, it seemed to me that the Ileal Conduit (Urostomy) might be my best option, so let me tell you a little bit about it. In this procedure, following the removal of the bladder, a conduit is created from leftover parts that will divert urine out of the body through a port (Stoma) which protrudes from my side. Attached to this port will be a reservoir (bag) which will need to be emptied as necessary. Are you ready for a really bad joke? This procedure will take the 'Pee' out of penis. Yes, that really was pretty bad and I should be embarrassed, but I am not. Let's blame it on chemo-brain.

At this point, I am picturing you, Dear Reader, saying to yourself, "This is the best option? That really doesn't sound so hot. Geez, how bad are the other options if this is the best?"

Please keep in mind that there is nothing too appealing about any of these choices. They all pretty much suck the big wazoo, with each having a few plusses to go along with a whole lot of minuses.

Think of it like the old, "Let's Make a Deal" game show when Monty Hall, the host, is offering a contestant, who's dressed in some zany costume, the choice between what's in the box, what's behind the curtain, or what's in the envelope he's holding. In the show, you could be sure that at least one of those options would be good and at least one would be ridiculously bad. (As I remember, they gave away a lot of farm animals on that show) Indulge me this fond memory. "Let's Make a Deal" was my father's favorite show, so much so that we nicknamed him, "*Marko* Make a Deal". Etched forever in my brain are images of him yelling at the television set in his broken English to, "Take the curtain! Take the CURTAIN!"

My situation is similar, except the gameshow I find myself playing would be named, "Let's Remove your Bladder", and all the options are pretty bad. But, when the bladder gotta go; the bladder gotta go. I'm picturing my father yelling, "Take the Ileal Conduit; take the ILEAL CONDUIT!" God bless him.

My doctor looked at my paperwork and went over my bullet points with me. He told me he was impressed that a patient would put that much work into researching their own options. (Well, someone has to do it, right?) I told him that beyond that, I had an opinion on which surgery I was leaning towards. When I told him that I thought the Iliad Conduit made the most sense for me, he was happy as that was going to be his recommendation.

You have heard me piss and moan about patient education and by now should know my feelings about doctors who chronically fail their patients when it comes to this important responsibility. I don't think I'm wrong in my opinions, and I feel that the medical community needs to be more aware of their shortfalls, but until each doctor makes the decision to change their behavior, don't expect to see meaningful improvement.

I believe I was fortunate to be researching bladder removal for several reasons. First, I understood pretty much everything I was looking at. Secondly, there were some very good websites for me to reference. Third, even more importantly, these websites all seemed to be saying the same thing. They were in accord with one another; they were singing out of the same hymnbook, which was reassuring for a layman trying to do his own research. You'll recall that when I described researching prostate screening on-line, the information was all over the board, and I came away more confused than educated.

When I went to see my doctor to discuss bladder removal, I was empowered with the greatest weapon of all: *information*. Yes, as a writer, I fully understand that that is a totally sappy statement, which I should be embarrassed about writing, but I'll let it stand as it does get the point across.

Let's talk for a moment about information. There has never been a better time in the history of the world to have a world of information literally at your fingertips. If you have access to the internet, you have access to information, and for better or worse, you have access to lots of information.

With a few clicks you can get to Web-MD, the New England Journal of Medicine, JAMA, and the American Cancer Society, along with numerous university sites like Harvard Medical and University of Chicago. You can drill down to individual hospitals like the Mayo Clinic, Sloan Kettering, and John Hopkins. There are even sites you can go to which will rate the best sites for you to reference for medical advice.

If you are inclined to venture into something weird, and who isn't, Google, 'Big Pharma Conspiracies' and you will be shocked, bewildered, and entertained at the accusations being hurled at the pharmaceutical manufacturers. According to many of these sites, big pharmaceutical companies have been playing fast and loose when it comes to our health. Apparently, there is a lot more money to be made by treating a disease as compared to curing a disease. There is a lot of smoke on these sites, but I'll leave it you to decide if there are fires raging behind them. All I'll say is that I hope most of what I read isn't true, because if it is, it's pretty scary to think their agenda could be so duplicitous and profit oriented.

Coincidently, as I write this, in the late summer of 2019, a huge story in the news deals with the Opiate Epidemic in the U.S. and big pharma's role in manufacturing and distributing mass quantities of these opiates. On that note; earlier this week (8-26-2019), an Oklahoma judge found Johnson & Johnson liable for the growing rates of opioid misuse and overdose deaths in the state. J&J was ordered to pay out $572.1 million in damages. Hmmm, maybe there is some fire to go along with all that smoke.

That's an interesting topic, but it's not really why we are here, so before we venture any further down that rabbit hole; let's move on.

My point is that information is available to you, and hopefully, with a little diligence on your part, you can find the answers you seek. That would be the ideal but it may not always work out that way as there are times the internet will answer your questions and other times you might walk away totally confused.

When I learned that I would be losing my bladder, it was encouraging to talk to people who either had their bladder removed or knew people who had lost their bladder. Through the friend of a friend, I ended up on the phone one morning with a total stranger who had lost his prostate and bladder in the same operation. This man was open and generous enough to discuss his operation with me, which I thought was incredibly kind of him considering he didn't know me from Adam. You can't have a meaningful discussion of these procedures without wading into some personal and private areas. I'll not share with you the finer points of this discussion, but I will say that he shared with me which of the three surgical options he chose and also told me of the good and bad of how he was recovering.

We were treated at different hospitals. When I told him how off-put I was over the lack of patient education prior to my prostate removal at my facility, he told me that he had the same experience at his hospital. The hospital he went to is considered one of the best in the country. Evidently, this discordant and out of tune song remains the same regardless of who's treating you.

One other option I wanted to bring to your attention, even though I have not taken advantage of these personally, is in-person support groups. I live in Chicago and found three groups that I would have access to. This may be a better option for those living near a large metropolitan area, as outside of the three in Chicago; I didn't see any other opportunities anywhere in Illinois.

I titled this chapter, 'So, what have I learned?' and reading back over it, I think I have learned a few things throughout my cancer journeys. To sum it up simply, let me say, "Knowledge is Power". I know that's a cliché, but I also see a lot of truth in it. I hope you might have gotten something worthwhile out of it as well.

Chapter Sixteen: Spinning wheels

I've walked you through my cancer experiences over the past thirteen or fourteen years, but I now find myself at the unenviable task of addressing the elephant in the room.

How is all this going to end?

This is not a new thought as it has nagged at me since I first took my cyber pen to my virtual paper and began writing *CANCER BABBLE*. I've done a good job of ignoring this inescapable issue over the summer, but the problem has really come home to roost over the last week. Even though I'm making good headway towards completing this book, I still don't know how this story is going to resolve itself. Now, how's that for a BIG elephant in the room. I'm a writer, and given the opportunity, I'm sure I could write a very satisfactory ending; an ending where I'm fine and the cancer is gone; an ending where I bask in eternal sunshine and rainbows shoot out of my butt. That would make for a wonderful finale. Who wouldn't like that ending?

As of this morning, I am about 43,000 words into *CANCER BABBLE*, and I'm very happy with my production so far, but I realized over the past week or so, that instead of soldiering on towards the finish line, I've been just spinning my wheels. I've been adding words to the story every day, because that's what a writer needs to do, but I'm not pushing the story towards its climax.

And now, once again, we are back to the elephant in the room.

What I've done instead of steering this story towards a conclusion is write about stupid things that people say, and chemo brain, and the Zen of writing. Objectively looking at my last several weeks of writing, it all just seems like so much filler.

Because I'm struggling with what to write next, I opted instead to print the manuscript and start my edits and rewrites. This is a safe way for me to feel like I'm making progress while not having to add to the story. I understand how to proofread this book; I just don't know how to finish it. I'm sorry, I know I'm repeating myself, but this is weighing heavily on my mind.

CANCER BABBLE

Writers are compelled to write, or at least they better be, or they'll never get a book on the shelf, which sadly happens all too often to aspiring, but less than inspired writers. I'm a writer, and yes, I'm compelled to write. That's not to say that writers don't get writer's block; we do. What I'm experiencing now can't be described as a block. It goes deeper than that. I sincerely want to finish telling you the story, but I can't. As I mentioned earlier (repeating myself, again), I'm not writing the end of this story. The universe is.

So, as long as I can't tell you everything, seeing as how I don't know everything, I can tell you this; I finished my chemotherapy yesterday. Much of my summer was spent in chemoland as my first three day course began on June 10, 2019, and my last three day course ended on August 28th. Let's see, June, July, and August; yep that's pretty much all summer by my way of thinking. I had bittersweet feelings about this milestone. Perhaps because I understood the chemo part of the treatment plan, I almost regretted leaving it behind. I came to know what to expect in chemoland, but I'm not too sure what to expect going forward. It's sad to think that chemo feels safe compared to whatever might be coming next.

I can also share this with you. Now that I finished my last barrage of chemo, I'll be going for a CT scan. This test has yet to be scheduled, but should be in the next two weeks. This scan will tell me if the cancer has spread. It will tell me if the copious amounts of chemo-poison they pumped through my system during this less than memorable summer of 2019 has done me any good. By my way of thinking, that makes it one scary goddamn test, wouldn't you agree? For those of you keeping score at home, yes, I'm already feeling angst about it. They sent me for a CT scan following the second round of chemo earlier this summer. At that time, there were small spots on my liver, but before anyone freaks out here, let me mention that these may be nothing to worry about. They may have been there for a while. This next scan will vet out just how concerned I should be about those little spots. I guarantee you that I am going to be pooping little green apples while waiting for the results of that test.

So, what else do I know? I know that the chemo beat the crap out of my blood, and that I'll need time to let it recover before the surgery to remove my bladder. That's really not a new thing. As a matter of fact, that's why I was given a twenty-day respite between each three-day chemo course. The second week following chemo is where my immune system would slump. Slump probably isn't the correct medical term, but I'm sure you get the point. The third week was when my system would start to recover; sometimes, but not always. Twice, I needed an extra week to bounce back from the chemo before I was ready to have more chemo-cocktail pumped into my system. Now that my chemo is complete, they want to give me several months for my system to repair itself before taking the bladder. On that note, my surgery is scheduled for November 7th, which will give me a 10-week rest and recuperation period.

I'm looking forward to this two month plus recovery time, and hope that I'll have an almost normal autumn. When you live in Chicago, fall is the season you live for. We enjoy temperatures in the mid-70s with low humidity. The nights are cool, and if you sleep with your windows open, at one point you'll pull the comforter over you and snuggle into its cocoon-like warmth. The skies are endlessly bright and blue and it's not uncommon to see flocks of birds, like Canadian Geese and Sandhill Cranes, hurrying on to some far distant places. Robins flee only to be replaced by the small yet sturdy Juncos. The hint of burning leaves scent the cool air, and at night the heavier fragrances of bonfires drift across the landscape. Pretty girls become even more beautiful as the cool fall air adds a natural blush to their cheeks. All of that takes a back seat to the explosion of colors as trees morph from green, to yellow, to red, to brown, and finally; to bare.

I promise you I will not take one moment of this upcoming season for granted. I'd be a fool not to savor each scent and every color that this autumn can offer me because when November does roll around; there will be changes in the air.

There will be changes in my life.

CANCER BABBLE

OK, I have come to a decision. I am going to shelve this book until I know more. Stopping a project like this is really out of character for me. I have trained myself to *'stay the course'* when writing. I have created production goals for my writing and stuck to those goals throughout my first four books. There is a law of physics that says, *'bodies at rest tend to stay at rest'*. That rule applies to writing. *Writers at rest tend to stay at rest.* In other words, there is an excellent chance that once I put this book to the side, I may never go back to it. This isn't my preferred approach as given my druthers, I would much rather keep on writing, but the troubling question remains, write what?

Cancer is an endlessly broad subject and I guess I could branch *CANCER BABBLE* off into some other directions. I'm sure I could write several thousand words on cancer research today, but that was never my agenda when I started writing. I could write even more on the history of cancer throughout the ages but, again, that was not my goal when I sat down to write. If you are interested in the history of cancer read, *The Emperor of All Maladies* by Sidhartha Mukherjee. It's an excellent book, but just so you know, it's very academic. Sidhartha is a lot smarter than me, but he's not nearly as funny.

I want to stay true to what I started out to accomplish, and even though *CANCER BABBLE* is all over the map as far as topics and subject matter go, it was never meant to deal with cancer history and research.

So on Saturday, August 31, 2019 at 9:53am, I am placing *CANCER BABBLE* to the side until I have more to share with you.

I hope to see you soon, Dear Reader, with good news.

Chris Drnaso

INTERMISSION

Let's all go to the lobby.

Chris Drnaso

Chapter Seventeen: An Update: Late September, 2019

For me, three weeks have gone by since I last wrote, whereas for you it is a simple turn of the page. I have been away, but I have not been idle. I worried when I set this project to the side several weeks ago that I might never get back to it. Well. I'm back. I spent my time doing a lot of edits and rewrites since last we spoke. There seems to be an unending amount of editing and proofing that goes along with writing a book. You may have been a victim of this yourself where it is difficult to catch your own mistakes. Thank God there are people in my life that are willing to read, proof, and comment on my work as, no matter how many times I go over my work, I still miss things. The brain works in mysterious ways. Have you ever seen that whole paragraph 'puzzle' where all the letters are jumbled, but you are still able to read it? In case you aren't familiar with what I'm describing, I've given you an example below.

I cnduo't bvleiee taht I culod aulaclty uesdtannrd waht I was rdnaieg. Unisg the icndeblire pweor of the hmuan mnid, aocdcrnig to rseecrah at Cmabrigde Uinervtisy, it dseno't mttaer in waht oderr the lterets in a wrod are, the olny irpoamtnt tihng is taht the frsit and lsat ltteer be in the rhgit pclae. The rset can be a taotl mses and you can sitll raed it whoutit a pboerlm. Tihs is bucseae the huamn mnid deos not raed ervey ltteer by istlef, but the wrod as a wlohe. Aaznmig, huh? Yaeh and I awlyas tghhuot slelinpg was ipmorantt!

Needless to say, spell-checker went nuts over that paragraph. Not everyone has the ability to read that paragraph, but there are many more who can than can't. I believe that the dynamics that allow you to read this jumbled up mess are the same dynamics that make it difficult to catch your own typos when proofreading. The brain sees what the brain wants to see.

My oldest friend in the world, who has read and commented on each of my first four books, gave *CANCER BABBLE* a read. Overall, he gave what I had written so far high grades. I asked him if he was just being kind to a cancer patient, and he assured me he wasn't. I held my breath when I asked him if I was really as goddamn funny as I thought I was, and he assured me that I am. Now, I'm really suspicious! We discussed the couple of chapters I wrote before going on hiatus, and we both felt they were weak. You, Dear Reader, may not see the worst of that as I'm trying to fix those chapters. It's what writers do. Part of the problem is chemo brain, but the bigger issue is not knowing how the book will end. My friend suggested that I write several endings to the book including one where I'm not around anymore. I have given that some thought, but in truth, I don't think I could do that. I feel I'd be tempting fate in a bad way.

I printed the book for Marilyn and asked her to read what I have written so far. She's not a reader, but because she loves me, she has somehow plowed through all of my books. One morning she told me she was close to finishing and asked that we hold off lunch until she was done. A short time later she closed the three-ring binder and placed it to the side. She was crying, and I thought, *"Christ, is it really that bad?"* Even I didn't realize that I shared emotions and feelings with you, my readers, which I never shared with her. It's not that I hide my feelings from her; it's more that I mask them in safer ways, often with humor. I love her dearly and it hurts to see how much this hurts her. I may be the one who is carrying these malignancies, but make no mistake; we are both going through cancer.

When we left off at the end of August, I made a point of how I wanted to enjoy the fall, and I'm happy to say that so far that game plan is falling into place. I have taken Abbey for lots of walks in the woods. She's old and slowing down. Her spirit is willing but the flesh is weak. What starts out as a walk turns into a drag as we find ourselves coaxing her along the myriad trails that we hike. What was once an easy walk for her is now more challenging. I understand and sympathize as I feel the same way on some of these walks. The chemo bombardment has taken its toll on me, and I find myself tiring easily, but I'm done with the chemo now and determined to build up some endurance and stamina before my November 7th date with the scalpel.

CANCER BABBLE

I'm excited to tell you that Marilyn and I took a ride to Michigan City, which on a good day is about an hour from the house. It was the first time I crossed a state-line in a very long time. How long? In truth, I can't remember; that's how long it's been. We had lunch at a little water front café and then walked the beach looking for pieces of driftwood for a craft project I've been thinking about. I was exhausted by the time we got home but it was a good fatigue.

On another day, we enjoyed brunch with friends.

We met up with some college friends for a very casual backyard get together.

I golfed! I have golfed for years, but I'm not a fanatic. I like golf. I don't love it, but I did find that I missed it as the last time I golfed I still had a prostate. That was about sixteen months ago. Many of my golf friends are purists, and we will forego a motorized cart and pride ourselves in walking the eighteen-hole courses we play. This time we played nine-holes, and at my request, we rode in a cart. That was probably the smart thing to do as even that was pretty exhausting. In case you are wondering, cancer has done nothing to improve my golf game.

My older son has been great about taking care of the yard work this summer. He shows up on Saturday morning with his laundry. Afterwards, he'll take a shower here before having lunch. This has made for some special bonding time. But now, I'm happy to announce, I am back to doing the yard work myself. It is a bit of a challenge, and I'll stop to take a break, but it is also very rewarding.

So, I jumped back into writing to catch you up on a few things that are going on. We talked about *CANCER BABBLE*, and I filled you in on some 'normal' things I've been doing this fall. Some of these activities may not seem like a big deal to you, but they have meant the world to me this autumn.

This update wouldn't be complete unless it included some medical mumbo-jumbo. As mentioned, I have completed my chemo and as planned, I was sent for a CT scan. Waiting for test results is always going to be a tense moment. The day after the scan, the caller ID displays my oncologist's name and, with great trepidation, I answer the phone. She is upbeat and cheerful on the phone, but that doesn't mean anything as she is always upbeat and exuberant. I like that about her. She is young and looks even younger. Marilyn and I agree that she could walk through any high school in the country and easily pass for a student; maybe even in a junior high.

That's enough about her. Let's get back to talking about what's really important; me. I know; I come across as a jerk when I say things like that. Mea Culpa. The news is good. The cancer has not appeared anywhere else and the spots on the liver appear to be cysts, which have not changed since previous scans. I'm sure that you, Dear Reader, have stressed over receiving news in your own lives. Maybe it was anxiously awaiting the birth of a child, or the fear of having a son or daughter in uniform that was stationed far from home. Perhaps, as with me, it was a test result. Hopefully that news, once delivered, has been good. News, like the Chicago weather, is unpredictable and not always good.

On that note, cancer is having a field day this summer with my friends. It is living proof that, *Cancer Never Sleeps*. I'm afraid to answer the phone as it seems like every time I do, I find out that someone else in my life has been afflicted. In the last week, I found out that two friends are dealing with skin cancer. A friend from high school sent a picture of the 10 internal and 35 external stiches it took to remove the cancer from his face. This morning, another friend is in Texas preparing for a two-day surgery. Her melanoma cancer is right near the eye, which makes for a tricky procedure. An old college friend in California has throat cancer. He was the guy we all wanted to be in college. Dudes wanted to hang with him, and chicks wanted to do him. Another friend has what they said was Stage IV liver cancer, but the good news is that he's actually doing really well at the moment. Another old friend, who has experienced unexplained weight loss over the past several weeks, went in for testing late last week. His wife called this morning. He has cancer at multiple places in his body. This one is really scary and not just because of the cancer, but because it came on so suddenly. He retired in the spring and was fully engaged in yard work, exercise, and even some travel when he realized he was losing weight. Yes, cancer is as unpredictable as a Midwestern tornado and just as cruel.

Cancer leaves it's victims with 'souvenirs'. You can't go through cancer without having emotional and physical reminders of your battle. We talked about chemo-brain, which can affect a person cognitively for many years. Of course there are the physical scars that serve as a very real reminder of treatments. Those never go away. A person can fight to get back to who they were before cancer and the lucky, or more determined, ones will come close, but I'm not sure if anyone makes it back from the edge of the abyss fully whole. I realize how dark these thoughts are, but they are one more reality of going through cancer.

One of the souvenirs that I have from my summer spent in chemoland is shortness of breath. I mentioned that I was blessed to have very few side effects from the chemo, but the breathing issues are both concerning and a little scary. Two flights, and a total of fourteen steps, will get you from my garage to the main living area of my home. Fourteen steps should not be a big deal for a guy who at one time climbed to the top of the 100-story John Hancock building, but I am sucking for air by the time I reach the top. I have been sent for several tests but there is no readily apparent reason for why I'm struggling. So, even though I am trying to avoid as many white coats as possible during this rest and recovery period, I am scheduled to go for a stress test.

Before we move on, let me mention that timing is everything. On that note, I am also scheduled for a colonoscopy during this brief recovery period. This doesn't have anything to do with my cancer; it's just the time to be retested. Really? My inclination is to blow it off but I live by the credo that if there is anything wrong, I want to be the first person to know about it.

In case you are wondering, if the doctor offers to let me watch the procedure on the monitor, I will politely tell him, "Thanks, but no thanks. Just wake me when it's over."

Chapter Eighteen: Did you hear about ...?

We have all been there. You run into someone or get a phone call and are told, "Did you hear about so and so?" You go on to find out that 'so and so' has cancer. The word cancer strikes a chord with people, perhaps because it is so prevalent. Remember, earlier in the book, when I made up the statistic that cancer, in one way shape or form, has affected close to 100% of the people on the planet. I don't care if I made that up; I believe it to be true. Feel free to prove me wrong if you wish. Regardless of the veracity of that statistic, the reality is that we have all received word that someone in our universe has cancer.

Because cancer is an ugly and cruel word, we can't help but be impacted by the news. Even when it's about someone that you are not all that close to; it still chills the spine.

You hear the news, and you want to do something. You feel you need to do something. So, what do you do?

You think to yourself that you'll make a phone call. A phone call is a great way to show you care. A phone call will show the world just how concerned you are. There's an intimacy to talking on the phone. In the words of an old Ma Bell advertisement: *'It's the next best thing to being there'*. But phone calls take effort, and you're a busy person, so you decide against it. Besides, maybe you'll be catching the patient at a bad time. You feel better about yourself once you convince yourself that calling the patient would actually be a huge imposition on the person. You're a caring sensitive person and certainly don't want to impose on anyone, especially someone who's sick. Upon further review, a phone call is definitely not the way to go.

Give yourself one gold star for avoiding making the call.

But you are caring and sensitive and you still want to do something. You decide to send a card. A card is an even better way of showing the patient just how concerned you are. Phone calls suck when compared to sending a card. You can picture the patient receiving the card and take delight when you think of how touched they'll be. Yep, a card is the way to go. You realize pretty quickly that the card actually takes more effort than the phone call. First, you have to go and get the card, and then fill it out and mail it. You haven't even bought the card yet, but you're already stressed over what to write. You're not even sure you have the right address even though this patient has lived in the same house for the past thirty-years. Another thing; stamps should not be that expensive. You blame ineptitude on the part of our political leaders for the price of stamps spiraling out of control. You are not going to endorse government inefficiency by buying stamps. There's another reason you are now not keen on sending the card. What are cards made of? Paper! You are at your core an environmentalist. You and Mother Earth are tight. You used to have a 'Save the Whales' bumper sticker on your car when you were in college for God's sake. You are not going to contribute to the deforestation of the planet by sending a card that is just going to end up in the garbage anyway. Knowing your friend, he probably won't even recycle the damn thing. You realize that there is no way, in good conscious, that you can send a card.

Congratulations, you get another gold star for not sending the card.

By this time, there have been multiple sunrises and sunsets since the day you first heard the sad news about so and so. Much of the worry and concern you felt upon hearing the news has faded. You realize at one point that it has been several days since you even thought about the cancer patient. Weeks go by and now you are struggling to even remember what type of cancer they had. Occasionally, it occurs to you that you never did make the phone call or send a card. In retrospect, you're not really sure why you didn't follow through on either of these things. Now, with so much time having passed, doing either of these things would seem awkward.

Oh my God! Why didn't you think of this before? You can send him a text. A text seems like the perfect solution. It's not as intrusive on the patient's time as a phone call would be. It is certainly more environmentally friendly than sending a card. You mull over all the things you want to say to the patient. You want to tell them that you prayed for them. You want them to know how the news of their trials has impacted you. You debate whether or not you should mention the unmade phone call or the unsent card. In your mind, this text keeps getting longer and longer. You realize that texts should not be long. Keep it short and to the point. Brevity, after all, is the nature of a text.

In the end, your text weighs in at four words. You text the patient, *"How are you doing?"* You climb into bed that night feeling wonderful about yourself. You bask in the glow of self-appreciation. You took the time out of your hectic life to reach out to a cancer patient to see how they're doing. Not everyone would be willing to do the same thing. You truly are a caring and concerned person. Your mother was right; you are a good boy. Dawn's first light finds you still giddy over just what a fine humanitarian you are. That little attention hound from Calcutta, Mother Teresa, has nothing on you. No sirree, Bob!

What do you say you get one more gold star? This time it's for being a complete douche bag.

OK, I realize that's harsh, but I don't believe it is undeserved. At this point, the patient has been dealing with cancer for weeks. In that time, he has had multiple doctors' visits. He has been sent for a barrage of tests and labs. There is an excellent chance that the patient has already been pulled into the world of radiation and chemotherapy. As mentioned earlier in the book, cancer patients lead very hectic lives, but the patient still has plenty of time on their hands to fret and worry over the disease. Time that a call or card or a visit from you might have helped him fill.

So, what is the expectation upon sending your four-word inquiry about the state of the patient's health? Did you imagine the patient would send you a two-thousand word update on their condition? A lot has been happening in their life and you did, after all, ask how they're doing. Would you even want some long winded explanation? It's likely you would want an even shorter reply. Perhaps something like, "I'm doing OK." That would close the book on this whole cancer thing nicely.

The only thing that can trump the insensitivity of a text is a Facebook posting. I'm rarely on social media even though Marilyn and I do have a Facebook page. We do nothing with this site even though people think it's

OK to post stuff on our page. I'd rather have you key my car as compared to posting something on my Facebook site. Just sayin'. One day, while I waited in a doctor's office, I thumbed through some Facebook pages on my phone. I stumbled onto one site that had posting after posting about cancer. The page belonged to someone I have known since the day she was born. Through three battles with cancer, she has never called me. She has never sent a card. She hasn't even sent the meaningless four-word, *'how are you doing?'* text. Nothing, zilch, nada, bupkis. But, and there's always a big but, she was able to find the time to make dozens of Facebook entries in an effort to show the world just how concerned she is about cancer. I can only speak for myself here, but as a cancer patient, your cancer-crusading Facebook postings mean less than nothing to me.

Keep in mind that I am dealing with some pretty serious chemo-brain, so perhaps you, Dear Reader, aren't too sure where your author is taking you in this chapter. That seems like a legitimate concern. (I know I'm a little concerned about it, too) Simply stated, there are meaningful ways to reach out to a cancer patient and, by contrast, there are some less than meaningful ways.

When I went through cancer for the first time in 2007, I told almost no one of what was going on. We told our sons, and I wanted to leave it at that. Marilyn put a gun to my head and demanded that I call my sisters. My wife is not a very demanding person, but I knew there was no debating whether or not I would call my siblings. When I did tell my sisters, I asked that they not say anything to my niece or nephews. With all that being said, I didn't hear from family or friends. How could I? They didn't even know I was sick.

Many months later, after I was finished with treatment and declared cancer free, we told family and friends of what we had been dealing with. Many of these people reached out to us with cards and calls or small gifts, and I realized at that time how meaningful these expressions of concern were. Many let me know they were upset at me for not saying anything, which in truth didn't bother me all that much. It was my cancer, so it was my business. What did strike a chord with me was when some people told me how unfair I had been to Marilyn by making her suffer in silence. I had denied her the right to a support group of her own, and I didn't realize how selfish that had been of me.

I can really feel the chemo-brain affecting me in this chapter. I believe I know what I'm trying to say but realize that I am struggling. You, Dear Reader, may never see this chapter, at least not in this incarnation. I may, with the help of friends, clean and clear a lot of it up before it ever gets to you. But, seeing how this is a book about dealing with cancer and all its side effects, I may leave it just as it is as a testimony on how cancer impacts cognition. As an author, I can't write nonsense and expect you to read it, so I am desperately trying to knit these thoughts together, so let's summarize. I started this chapter by talking about how family and friends can drop the ball when it comes to reaching out to a cancer patient. Re-reading the first few paragraphs of this chapter, I can see that I really portrayed this person as a complete dick. There's a temptation to either eliminate that section or at least to soften it a bit, but I don't think I want to do that, so I'll leave it stand.

Instead, I believe I'll ask you, the reader, this question instead. "Did you recognize yourself in those first couple of paragraphs?" Are you the guy who thinks about calling, but doesn't? Did it cross your mind to send a card, but ultimately, you couldn't be bothered? I'm not interested in being your Father-Confessor, and I sure as hell ain't your moral compass, but what I came to understand over multiple battles with cancer is that a phone call or a card can turn a cancer patient's shit-day into a pretty good day.

What you do is ultimately your decision, but I will ask you to not dangle shiny objects in front of a cancer patient and then snatch them away. Please explain, you ask. OK, for starters, never contact a cancer patient and offer to do something for, or with them, and then blow them off. Let's start with a happy story. When I was going through my second battle with cancer, a friend called and asked if I felt well enough for him to stop over with a couple of sandwiches and just hang out. He brought his dogs, and while they frolicked in the yard with Abbey, he and I sat on the deck and ate and talked. It was a wonderful afternoon and it meant a lot to me that he would do this.

Alright, you should know me well enough by this time to know what's coming. My friend happened to mention this visit to a mutual friend of ours. Upon hearing how much I appreciated the visit, and how rewarding it was for our friend to extend such a thoughtful kindness to a cancer patient, I received a call from this mutual friend. He, too, wanted to pick up some sandwiches and come a calling. I was thrilled as I had a lot of long days while recovering from my surgery. There is a limit to the amount of alone time I can deal with so being able to sit and talk to someone for a couple of hours was wonderful to look forward to. He committed to giving me a call in a couple of days to secure a date. Days went by and no call. Days turned into weeks and still no follow up. So much time went by that I had actually survived my second cancer and was now battling my third cancer before I heard from this guy again. You may not believe this, and even though I can spin a yarn, I am not making this up. I ran into this old friend and the first thing he said was that he had heard that I was once again going through cancer. He asked if it would be OK to pick up some sandwiches and stop by for a visit. He had a good deli in his neighborhood and even asked me what kind of a sub I wanted. He was busy over the next few days but would call me to set up a good date for our lunch. As Yogi Berra is credited with saying, "*It was like Déjà vu all over again.*" Days became weeks and then months and still no call.

To give you an idea of how I felt about all this, I am going to drop the F-bomb for the first time in this book when I ask the rhetorical question, "Who the FUCK does this to anyone, let alone a cancer patient?"

If you don't want to send me a card; fine, I'm OK with that. If you don't call, I can live with that, too. Truthfully, I'd rather you didn't send me a meaningless four word text, but heed my words, DON'T DO THIS. Please don't ever do something like this to a cancer patient. We're dealing with enough crap of our own, so we sure don't need any of yours.

Wow, I just reread that last section and evidently your author is dealing with some unresolved anger issues. Well, in truth, it felt good to get it out.

Chris Drnaso

In 2006, I received word that my cousin was dealing with cancer. As happens all too often, after childhood we had drifted apart, and in truth, I rarely saw him even though we had been fiercely close as kids. I called him. I'm not sure why, but it took a lot of courage for me to make that phone call, and to this day, I don't know why I felt so much trepidation. We had made each other laugh so much as kids, and after a brief moment on the phone, we found ourselves laughing once again about everything and anything. I received so much by making a simple phone call. We both did. After that first call, we kept in touch regularly. One day Marilyn and I left soup on his front porch; another day we stopped by with ice cream.

Life can throw some funny things at you and several months later, it was me who was fighting cancer. This time my cousin called me, and once again, we laughed. I really needed that. It wasn't long after that, when my cousin lost his battle with cancer. We buried him on a blustery late winter day. His family had welcomed me into their inner circle, and I was with him when he passed. It hurt, and I wept. I was one of six who was honored with carrying his casket. There has been so many times when I think about what I would have lost if I had not made a simple phone call to someone who was going through a bad patch. For me, it was the essence of *'bread cast upon the water'*.

I learned from the experience with my cousin. I'm not trying to be a harbinger of bad tidings, but I can pretty much guarantee you that a day will come when the phone will ring and you will be told that someone you know has cancer. I hope when that day comes you think back to a silly little book called *CANCER BABBLE* and a chapter labeled, *'Did you hear about …?'*

Chapter Nineteen: Maybe I did too good of a job?

Today's date is Tuesday, October 29, 2019: I gave you an update in late September. At that time, I told you I was going to embrace every minute of the beautiful Chicago fall weather, and I did; I really did. As a matter of fact, I did this to such an extent that on most days I was able to put cancer out of my head completely. Poof, and just that easily the dark thoughts were gone. Part of it was that I felt good. Week after week, the fatigue that accompanied my chemo was less of a factor. Physically, I felt stronger, and I refused to let any of the little chronic things that go along with cancer bother me. I ignored the back pain, and the shortness of breath, and my limited stamina. I didn't let any of that get in the way of all that I wanted to do during this fall season. It felt wonderful to complete some household task and not be wiped out by it. Even my hair started to slowly grow back in. It wasn't as thick and black (except for the stuff growing out of my nose and ears; what's up with that?) as I hoped it might be, but you take what you can get. As I mentioned earlier, there were walks and golf and yardwork and day-trips out of state with Marilyn. All this made it so easy to forget about the cancer. I don't know if it's fair to say that I forgot about the cancer, but I certainly didn't dwell on it. I did a good job of burying the disease in the far recesses of my mind, but maybe I did too good of a job.

One thing that helped me forget was that I had less white coat time during this nine-week respite. I mentioned that I was scheduled for a colonoscopy, and (are you ready for another one of Chris' childish jokes?) I'm happy to say that everything came out OK. Those of you who have prepped for a colonoscopy in the past will get the joke. For those who haven't had the pleasure, let me just say that you are in for a big surprise down the road. The results were great. No polyps. After the procedure the doctor told me that I didn't need another colonoscopy for ten years. The idea of being vertical for another ten years is enchanting and wonderful to think about, but I'm not all that sure I'm going to be around six months from now. Think good thoughts, I remind myself.

I mentioned that my doctor retired, and I told you of the high opinion I had of the man. I was able to become a patient of record with one of his associates from his same medical team. I go for an annual physical every October and so I had my first visit with my new doctor recently. It was a great first meeting. I told her of the respect I had for my doctor who had retired and that she had big shoes to fill. I feel really good about this relationship as she seems to be cut from the same cloth as my former doctor. I sleep better at night knowing I have a good doctor. She was also very punctual during this first encounter, and I hope that is the norm and not the exception.

Because I was complaining of shortness of breath, I was given a stress test. This was what is known as a nuclear stress test which means an injection simulates your body exercising. I could have sat through the whole thing or slowly walked a treadmill for four minutes. I opted to walk the treadmill because, as I mentioned, I am feeling good. The whole process was pretty exhausting. It took about three and a half hours as there is a lot of waiting around between tests. I was dreading this test but, in truth, it wasn't all that bad. The fact that it was a rainy crappy day made it very tolerable to just sit and read a book.

These white coat visits were scattered throughout my nine-week rest and recuperation period so it never felt like too much of an infringement on my time, which was good as I had a lot to pack in during this interval. I drifted through this period in a state of blissful delusion. Stated as an axiom; *if I'm feeling this good, and I'm being this active, then I can't be all that sick*, right? One must be careful with axiomatic logic as oft times it will lead you away from the truth you seek.

The reality of my situation all came crashing in on a recent Monday morning when Marilyn and I made the trip to the hospital for a pre-surgical consultation. Delusion and denial tend to fly out the window when you are shown the mechanics of living without a bladder. You can't pretend any longer that there is nothing wrong when they show you the bag that will become part of your body for the remainder of your life. Only a fool will continue to believe that everything is fine when they take a magic marker and place a dot on your belly to map out where the tube (stoma) will exit the body. This is a difficult consultation to get through. I'm trying to be stoic, and

I remind myself that there are thousands of people in the world who have gone through this procedure, and if you believe the hype, they are living full and active lives with this device protruding from their side. In truth, this knowledge offers little comfort.

Maybe if I felt sick, or was in pain, it might help to make this surgery seem vitally essential, but I don't feel sick and there is no pain. I keep waiting for some voice of reason to step in and say, *"There must be some mistake here. You look good and feel strong. You're being active and your hair's growing back in. We double checked the records and it turns out you are absolutely fine. What do you say we quit all this nonsense about cancer and your bladder and let you get back to living a long and healthy life?"*

But no one has said this, and I'm not expecting an eleventh hour call from the governor granting my bladder a full pardon. The die has been cast; the jury has spoken, and the execution of this organ will go on as scheduled.

Believe me, Dear Reader, when I tell you, that I did an exemplary job of forgetting about my cancer over this multi-week rest period. It turns out that if you can manage to get the cancer thoughts out of your head, you just might be able to keep the dark thoughts that accompany cancer at bay, too.

Now, those dark thoughts are back, and they are here to stay. No matter how hard I try to be brave, this is a difficult hit to absorb.

We have a dear friend who was completely blind-sided by cancer this summer. I mentioned him earlier in the book when I spoke of how we hesitated to answer the phone lest we discover that yet another friend has been diagnosed with cancer. Our friend's wife asked Marilyn if I would be interested in meeting with her brother who is a Catholic priest. She invited us to her home where her brother would bless both her husband and me. I was interested, but I know me, and I know I would have a tough time getting through this emotionally. Full disclosure here; I have wept many times over these past months, but I shed most of these tears in private moments when no one else is around. Marilyn will occasionally find me sobbing quietly, but I try to spare her this pain as she has her own difficult moments as well. Many people consider me the poster child for cancer. I'm the guy who absorbs these challenges with a spring in his step and a smile on his face; the guy who laughs at cancer. The truth is that I am very good at pretending that I'm handling things well. Our friend's wife wanted me at the blessing because I'm dealing with cancer so well, and her husband draws strength from my stoicism. Well, that's two people I've done a good job of fooling. When I called my friend's wife to discuss her offer, I broke down almost immediately. So much for my fragile façade of the guy who looks cancer in the face and laughs.

Our friend is so sweet. She and her brother visited us in our home that morning. I handled this arrangement marginally better, but believe me; I shed many tears that morning. He assured me this wasn't the Last Rites, even though from my vantage point there wasn't a great deal of difference. He and I sat on our deck where he heard my confession in private. Following that, we went back in the house and sat with Marilyn and our friend. He said some prayers before anointing my head and hands with oil. We received communion. I mentioned that I am blessed to see signs of God all around me every day. On that morning, sitting in my living room, I felt His presence lift my spirit and feed my soul.

Her brother, the priest, took a liking to Abbey, but that's not unusual, because as Marilyn says, "Everyone likes Abbey." It's true, too. Anyway, as we sat in a loose circle, Abbey joined us and watched the proceedings with rapt attention, so much so that the priest commented on how the dog seemed to be captivated and engaged by these events. That all sounds rather ecclesiastical but the reality is that Abbey saw the priest feed me a communion wafer, and she was hoping he might have a treat for her as well. An important life lesson: Things aren't always what they seem.

God bless our friend and her brother for taking the time to do this for both Marilyn and me.

Halloween has come and gone. This is a big day in the Drnaso house. I have always loved Halloween. When we were kids, we didn't have a great deal and that meant there was rarely candy in the house. Halloween was the day my sisters and I could remedy that. Like sugar craving street urchins, we trudged the neighborhood on a quest to get enough candy to last for the rest of the year. We never met that goal, but it wasn't for lack of effort. This year it snowed in Chicago on Halloween. I'm not talking about a few flurries; there was an actual snow storm; a blizzard that left several inches of snow behind. Chicago can have some pretty raw weather but snow on October 31st is out of the norm. Chicago kids are cut from strong stock and over fifty trick or treaters braved the elements and rapped upon my chamber door. I'm so proud of them. Such is the depth of my despair over my upcoming surgery that the site of ghouls and goblins actually lifted my spirits. (No pun intended)

This may seem like a strange question, but do you have a tree that you love? I think most people do, and there are several trees that I look forward to watching in the spring or fall. We have a chestnut tree in our yard that has helped us mark the passage of time over the thirty-seven years that we have been in our home. It was here when we moved in, but it was just a baby at that time. Now, it is a huge and powerful specimen. I love that tree; Marilyn does, too. It is unpredictable. It bears fruit, but there is no rhyme or reason to whether you will get a few chestnuts or a bushel full. It doesn't make any difference as the nuts are poisonous and therefore inedible. In the fall, as its leaves begin to change, you would think this tree was diseased or dying as the broad green leaves turn a sickly brown. Then, several days before it drops its leaves, it turns a lovely golden-yellow color. It is beautiful, but it almost appears that the effort of putting on this late fall display is too much, and it will then drop all of its foliage in a single morning over the course of several hours. This year, it was the day after Halloween that our lovely chestnut tree decided it was time to turn the page from autumn to winter, and I watched as the leaves began to drop. As I watched, mesmerized by the display, there was never a time that thirty or fifty or a hundred leaves weren't drifting down at the same time. And then, by noon, the show was over. The canopy, that had shaded and cooled us over the summer, now rested on the ground. No longer did these leaves look down upon the yard from their lofty perch. Instead they lay on the ground and looked up at the

147

sky through the bare branches above. Several years ago, when this annual show was over, I noticed that one leaf clung fiercely to its perch. The next day, and for several days after that, it still hadn't fallen. I cheered for this leaf and encouraged it to hang on for as long as possible.

I'm not a poet, but occasionally the muses speak to me, and I'll be inspired to write a poem. I wrote the following poem years ago as a tribute to this determined little leaf.

The Last Leaf of Autumn
Autumn 2009
By Chris Drnaso

See the tree standing there
Once so lush but now quite bare

All its leaves are gone save one
A lonely leaf in the autumnal sun

It's time to go has long since passed
And yet its grip is strong and fast

Alas, you ask, *"Why does it wait?"*
When all the others did not hesitate

To leave their perch and seek the ground
Only to be raked and bound

Could it be that our lone leaf
Aspires to the strong belief

That the joy that comes with each new day
Justifies his long delay

But now his strength grows weak and weary
As the days get shorter; the weather dreary

Then one day, our lone leaf fell
But there was one who saw and wished him well

For what he learned from this last leaf
Is to seize each day as life is brief

CANCER BABBLE

I warned you that I'm not a poet, but I've always liked that poem. I actually think it's pretty good for an admitted non-poet. If I didn't feel that way, I would never have included it. Lately, I feel a lot like that leaf.

It's Sunday morning; November 3rd, and now just days before my surgery. I'm writing as I wait for my sons to come over and help with the fall yard work. I'm trying to get everything done so Marilyn won't have to worry about any of this. As I write, she's in the other room sewing. This is typical and especially comforting today as I've cried several times this morning. This surgery scares me. The doctors have pulled no punches. This is a difficult surgery. There will be pain, something I'm not a big fan of. There will be five to seven days in the hospital following the surgery, some of that time in intensive care. They told me it would be weeks before I felt OK and up to six months before I would start to feel like my old self again. Will I ever feel like my old self again?

I've spent a lot of time in *CANCER BABBLE* talking about patient education. Today, a scant two-days before my surgery, I decided to 'man-up' and research mortality rates for the surgery I'm about to go through. Of course, my research led me to the internet and, of course, the data I retrieved was inconsistent between different sites. The mortality rate for bladder removal surgery (cystectomy) ranges from concerning to insignificant depending on the site I'm on. For instance, I love the Mayo Clinic site which states, *'Rarely, death can happen after surgery'*. Who wouldn't love that? Another site showed a mortality rate of between .8% and 8%. I only feel good about one of those numbers. (Guess which one) One site showed a person's five year survival rate at 77 percent. I'm not sure how I feel about that one.

It's more than the mortality rates that have me knotted up. If you have general good health before the operation, one major complication will still affect 25 to 30% of patients after their surgery. These complications include infections, blood clots, heart attack, or stroke. Beyond that there are hernias, kidney stones, and obstructions to worry about. And of course we can't forget about the biggest concern of all, and that's the chance that cancer, that most devious and untrustworthy of all adversaries, will show up uninvited and unannounced somewhere else.

One morning this week, I penned a letter to my wife. It was a goodbye letter. It was very personal, so you can see why I might hesitate to print it. I've sent it to a trusted friend and asked him to deliver the letter to Marilyn in case things go badly on Thursday during my surgery. I debated whether or not I would share this with you, and then I realized that if I don't make it through the surgery, this book will never be published anyway, so I may as well post it here.

Thursday, October 31, 2019

My Dearest Marilyn,

I hope you never receive this letter as that would mean that my November 7th, surgery to remove my bladder went well. If you are reading this, then maybe things didn't go as we hoped.

Wow, this is harder to write than I thought it would be. My thoughts are scattered, and I'm not sure where to start.

I am the luckiest guy in the world to have found you all those years ago. Having you in my life made my life worth living. There was never a time that I was with you that I wasn't happy just to be near you. You lit up a room whenever you walked into it; you lit up my heart when you walked into my life. I drew strength from just holding you close and breathing in your essence.

When I first saw you, I didn't know who you were, but I thought you were beautiful, and every day since then, you somehow became more beautiful. It's remarkable that in all the years we have been together there has hardly been a harsh word between us. I don't think too many couples can make that claim.

I remember many times that we told each other that we wanted to be the first to go, as the thought of going through life without each other was too heartbreaking to even think of.

Now, I'm gone, and I am so sorry to have left you. The time we had together was not enough. A millennium wouldn't have been enough time. But you are not alone. I will always be with you; in memories and pictures and in your heart. There are a thousand little things all around you that will remind you every day of our journey together. I know you see parts of me in Matt and Nick. Please remind the boys often that their father loved them and no one will ever have their best interest in heart as much as I did. If they are happy, then they are rich.

Marilyn, I want you to find happiness without me in your life. Right now that probably doesn't seem possible, but there will come a day, hopefully soon, that you will find a reason to smile. We shared so much laughter in our life, and I want you to find something to laugh about each day. I don't know where I'll be once I walk through the veil to the other side, but I hope I can still hear the sound of your laughter. Then I'll know I'm in heaven.

It seems like I should have some deep or profound way to end this short note, but as I ponder this, I can't think of a better way than simply to say; I love you. I always have, and I always will. ...Chris

Today's date is November 5th, 2019. It is two days before my surgery and I have once again set *CANCER BABBLE* to the side. I hope the story has engaged you up to this point and that you are anxious to read the ending. I know I am. Wish me luck!

Chris Drnaso

Post-Surgery

Chris Drnaso

Chapter Twenty: I'm back...finally

Sunday, March 29, 2020:

Yes, that date is correct.

It has been close to five months since my surgery. Of course for you, Dear Reader, through the miracles of modern science, it was simply a matter of turning the page and, *'Viola!'* you have fast-forwarded through this long absence and have been delivered into the here and now.

I didn't plan on this long of a hiatus...it just happened. When I went into surgery on November 7th, 2019, I envisioned being back on the keyboard within a few weeks. I actually thought about bringing my laptop with me to the hospital and writing the next morning. Needless to say, that didn't happen.

So, what did happen?

"Where the hell has this guy been for the past five months?" you may rightfully ask.

Let's table that for a moment and talk first about what I hoped might happen. What I hoped for was a miraculously quick recovery. I mentioned that I went into this surgery feeling strong. I had exercised throughout the fall. I had intentionally gained weight as I was told that I could expect to lose weight following the surgery. This led me to believe that I would be out of that hospital bed so soon and on my way home that my recovery would become the stuff of legends.

Things actually did get off on the right foot. I was told that I could expect to spend 5-to7 days in the hospital following the surgery. I was told no one leaves before the five-day mark. (Stay tuned for *'Chris' Tips on how to get out of the hospital'*, coming soon to a chapter near you) I wanted to go home as soon as possible, which probably describes everyone who has ever been in the hospital for any reason. I am happy to announce that I did leave the hospital after the minimum five days. Did I feel good? No, not really, but I figured that I would rather feel lousy at home instead of feeling lousy in the hospital.

So now my post-surgical chronicle has begun and this is where I'm struggling with what to write. I mentioned at the beginning of this chapter that I wanted to be the poster child for what a full and quick recovery looks like. I wanted you, my Dear Readers, to marvel at the tenacity and stoicism of your author. That was of paramount importance to me. I'm a writer, and I guess I could just lie to you. Most of you would never know the difference, but I have tried to be forthright up to this point, and I would disappoint myself if I were to misrepresent my experiences.

My guess is that most of you have intuited by this time that there may have been issues with my recovery.

You're right, and that's part of the reason that five-months have elapsed before I started writing again. *'Part of the reason'* is the key phrase in that last sentence. There were actually a collection of reasons that kept me off the keyboard.

I spoke earlier in the book about 'chemo-brain' and the effect it had on cognition and how this could affect a person for weeks or months or years. Cognitive impairment was a huge issue over this five-month period and it went well beyond the effects of the chemo I had been exposed to. I wasn't prepared for the way my cognition dropped off. For example, I have always enjoyed crossword puzzles, and even though I was never going to be one to complete the *New York Times* puzzle in ink, I considered myself pretty good at these brain teasers. For probably four months following my surgery I couldn't even complete easy puzzles. This was both amazing and concerning as I would stare at the clues without a clue as to what the answers might be.

Several friends had dropped off books after my surgery as they knew I was an avid reader and thought books might help to fill my recovery time. This was a lovely gesture and, under other circumstances, would have been much appreciated. Like the puzzles, the books also seemed alien and unknowable to me. They would mockingly sit on my head board, reminding me that I was now a mere shadow of the man I had once been.

There were frightening aspects to this as I didn't know when, or if, my mental functions would come back. During this period I would pick up a puzzle or a book, stare at it silently for a moment, and then set it back down dejectedly as I realized that it was beyond my abilities.

You could imagine that if reading and puzzles had stymied me this greatly, the thought of writing was certainly way beyond my capabilities.

As you can see, I have started writing. Approximately four months after my surgery, I picked up a crossword puzzle and, I am happy to say, completed it without an issue. I didn't question what had happened, I was just glad that it had happened. My next thought was that if the ability to complete puzzles had returned, maybe I should try reading. That evening when I climbed into bed; I read. It was a bit of a struggle but I made it through the introduction of a book my son had dropped off. A week or so later, I had finished that book and started another. I felt like a person who had lost something precious and who feared the loss might be permanent, but now, this priceless gift had been returned to me.

Reading and puzzles, along with a LOT of TV, were a godsend during this period as I was under 'house arrest' for weeks at a time. My immune system had been greatly compromised following my surgery. Weight loss and fatigue exacerbated the situation. I was now considered anemic and warned by my medical team to avoid crowds or anyone who wasn't feeling well. I was already used to this isolation from my summer in chemoland as the same rules applied during that period.

I just realized that I have gotten way ahead of myself here. Somehow, I took you from my surgery and fast forwarded you five months into the future. That wasn't my intention so let's turn the clock back.

The date is November 12th and it has been five days since my surgery. I am now home. Somehow, I am able to navigate the fourteen steps that take me to the living quarters of our home. I plop on the sofa, exhausted from the effort. I guess this is to be expected. I focus on a singular thought; I am home now and my goal is to feel a little bit better every day. Baby steps, I tell myself. I take a real shower. A warm shower is always good medicine. I'm careful as I bathe as the reality of being surgically altered is staring me in the face. There is a bag attached to my side. I hate the bag already. It scares me, and I don't want it, but it is now and forever a part of my anatomy. For the next several days Marilyn and I watch the bag suspiciously; waiting for it to fall off or explode or spontaneously combust but that doesn't happen. Instead, it leaks. Together we try to remember all the instructions we received in the hospital on the care and feeding of an ileostomy bag. We manage to change the device but aren't entirely sure we have correctly completed the procedure. As it turns out, we will have many, many more chances to improve our technique as the bags will continue to fail (leak). They may last a day or, best case, as many as five days, but you can bet the rent that at some point they will fail.

Thanksgiving is right around the corner. Marilyn and I traditionally host the holiday for the family. The day is meaningful for both of us as, even though we give thanks daily for all the blessings bestowed upon us, there is something special in the thanks we offer on this special day. This year the family scrambles to make other plans. Thanksgiving is late this year and I hold onto the unrealistic hope that I may be able to at least make an appearance at the dinner.

That hope is dashed during the prior week. Shortly after getting up I am brushing my teeth when I tell Marilyn that I have a blood clot in my leg. She wonders how I can be so sure and all I can say is that I had a blood clot following cancer treatment in 2007 and there is a very distinct sensation that accompanies a clot. There is numbness in my right calf; it feels like my leg has fallen asleep. The calf is swollen. I'm not a doctor and there is always the hope that I am wrong about the clot. I engage my medical team. The medical community takes a blood clot very seriously. My home care nurse is scheduled to visit that day. She agrees that it sounds like a clot, and as my nurse completes the exam, Marilyn prepares to take me to the hospital.

I'm not making this up. Marilyn passes out right in front of me and the nurse. I call 911 as the nurse tends to Marilyn. That day Marilyn and I go to the hospital in separate ambulances, ten-minutes apart. How's that for a day that will live in infamy? Normally, a blood clot would not be a reason to call an ambulance, but as I mentioned, the medical community take a blood clot seriously and there was no one else available to take me to the hospital, so that is how I got my first ride ever in an ambulance.

I mentioned throughout this book that it is not only the patient who goes through cancer. The caregiver is right there in the trenches every step of the way with the patient. The caregiver must deal with the stress and responsibilities of looking after the patient. At first I thought that Marilyn had succumbed to the inherent pressures of being a caregiver. I thought she had been overwhelmed by the moment. I was wrong.

It turns out that she was much more focused on taking care of me instead of herself. She wasn't eating well. Her sleep, which was erratic, was not doing enough to recharge her batteries. Tests in the hospital showed that she had mineral and vitamin deficiencies. I felt terrible, as I knew it was my condition that was directly responsible for her predicament.

For all you cancer patients out there, please treat your caregivers well as they are doing so much for you and going through more than you can imagine. They need your support. It's a two-way street.

As for me, I was right; ultrasounds showed that I had developed blood clots in my leg, which then moved their way into my lungs, which made a bad situation worse. For the next week I was in the hospital as they pumped blood thinners into me.

Marilyn was in a room two floors below me dealing with her own issues. At one point a sympathetic nurse 'wheel-chaired' her up to my room for a short visit. It was wonderful to spend a few moments together even though there was something surreal about the whole situation. On that Saturday night, I called her to tell her I had found *Forrest Gump* on TV. It's one of our favorite movies, and she tuned it in immediately. There was something comfortable, almost conspiratorial, about sharing the same movie while being separated by several floors. At the end of the movie, while the credits rolled, I called her room to ask if she was crying. She was, but I knew that even before I dialed the phone.

Several days later Marilyn was released from the hospital, and a few days later I followed her home. This was at the beginning of Thanksgiving week and I knew that there was no way I would be joining the family for the holiday. Instead, our daughter-in-law showed up at our home early on that Thursday morning with a turkey along with all the fixings in tow. She proceeded to prepare a beautiful Thanksgiving meal for Marilyn, and me, and our two sons.

This will always be one of my most memorable Thanksgivings. Certainly, one of the most unforgettable.

There are truly special moments that I experienced while going through cancer. (Nothing's all bad, right) Thanksgiving was one of those moments. On a Saturday morning in early December, Marilyn and I were sitting in the living room. The mood that morning was somber; quiet, and we were saying little to one another. The doorbell rang and right on the heels of that we heard singing. There were Christmas carolers in our driveway. As Marilyn headed for the front door, I called for her to bring her wallet as oftentimes carolers will also collect for some charity.

That wasn't the case. What we found were a dozen friends standing in our driveway all singing Christmas songs. As Marilyn opened the door one friend walked in carrying a huge basket of goodies. There were blankets and cookies and fruit. There was homemade soup. There were sketchbooks and colored pencils. It was an amazing collection of all sorts of things.

Marilyn and I were overwhelmed by the moment and tears flowed freely to think that our dear friends would take the time to do something so special for us.

We invited them in, but they refused as they had other stops to make on this morning. I mentioned that cancer had been rough on our friends during this year. They had already visited one friend who was dealing with cancer, and after leaving our home, they needed to visit another friend who was also fighting cancer.

I freely admit that I am not a good enough writer to describe how wonderful this gesture was and how much it meant to both of us. It is not an exaggeration when I say that neither Marilyn nor I will ever forget this special morning. Our friends started out that morning to sing a few songs and drop off some goodies, but they gave us more than they will ever know.

Chapter Twenty-One: The Journey Continues

My encouragement at getting released from the hospital a scant five-days after my surgery is short lived as I find myself back in the hospital thanks to the blood clots. I felt them in my legs initially before they decided they could make my life more miserable by moving to my lungs. I am unprepared for how these clots have impacted my breathing. Even simple efforts have me sucking for air like a man trying to breathe with a plastic bag over his head.

I have more fight in me, and I'm not going to let this setback derail me on my road to recovery. I will get through this. With Thanksgiving behind me, I set a new goal of spending Christmas with the family. That gives me about a month to heal. I think I can do this, even though the clots are impacting me greatly. As it turns out, it seems the ability to breathe is pretty important to a person's overall well-being; who knew? As mentioned, there is nothing normal about my breathing. They assign me an in-home physical and occupational therapist who slowly and cautiously guide me on my path to wellness. Marilyn borrowed a walker from a friend following my surgery and I continue to use it. I don't feel good about depending on it but there is no doubt that I need it as I am pretty shaky on my feet. I envision a day when I won't need the walker anymore, but I suspect that day is still a ways off.

In other news, when they removed my bladder they also took a goodly amount of lymph tissue as well. They then sent all of this for a biopsy. Somewhere between Thanksgiving and Christmas, I meet with my oncologist to learn the results of the tests.

Drumroll please...you are in the presence of someone who has now heard, for the third time in his life, that he is cancer free. None of that makes me smart or good looking, but it does make me one of the luckiest son-of-a-bitches you'll ever meet.

The news is wonderful but it comes with some surprises. My oncologist tells me that they saw no evidence of cancer in the bladder or the lymph tissue.

Hmmm, that's good, but it begs the question, "So why did you remove my bladder?"

I know there was cancer in my bladder in the spring. I had a non-invasive surgery and a tumor was removed. It was cancerous. That was the catalyst for months of chemo as well as the surgery to remove the bladder.

I am told that if they had not removed the bladder, there was a 50% chance that the cancer would return. But, now that they have removed the bladder, there is only a 30% chance the cancer would come back.

In truth, I believe both of those percentages SUCK big time, but all a guy can do is to be grateful that, for today at least, the cancer is gone. Going forward, every so often, my oncologist will send me for a scan to determine if the cancer is behaving itself or if it has crept back in *'on little cat feet'* like Carl Sandburg's *Fog*. For anyone that has gone through this, it is a stressful moment as you wait to hear the results of the scan. If the news is good, you go out and celebrate; if it's not good, then your life is about to get turned upside down.

My job at the moment is to get better. I take inventory. The removal of my bladder is behind me, which was the biggest hurdle to get over. The clots in my lungs are impacting me greatly, but I focus on the fact that they are being managed by the blood thinners. At some point, this too shall be little more than a distant and unwelcome memory. Even though I get exhausted quickly, I try to walk in the house every day. I'm amazed at how winded I get by doing so little. Chicago, in 2019, is blessed to have one of the mildest December's on record, which actually allows me to walk outside with my physical therapist on one particularly warm day. I don't walk far, and I am still dependent on the walker, but neither of those things diminishes the wonderful feeling of being off the couch and out of the house for a few moments.

My entire family is cheering for me to make an appearance on Christmas day. (Perhaps they do like me more than I thought). Christmas morning, like much of December, dawns with freakishly mild weather. The day starts with our daughter-in-law (God bless her) making breakfast for our family. After that, a few gifts are exchanged. We sip coffee while Christmas carols play in the background. There is an excitement in the air because I am feeling good and will be making the trip to my sister's house to join the rest of the family for our Christmas celebration. I warn my sister that I may not last long, but she, along with the rest of the family, understands. They are just happy to learn that I'll be with them. It is a wonderful day for me. Before dinner, I ask if anyone would like to take a walk with me. Many in the family join me on my twenty-minute, walker assisted trek. Ok, I may have been bragging a bit when I claimed the walk was twenty-minutes, but regardless of how long it actually lasted, I was still able to get a walk in that day.

Being with the family in such a convivial setting energizes me. I went from not knowing how long I'd be at the party to not wanting to leave. The sun has been down for hours by the time Marilyn and I return home.

I climb into bed that night believing that the worst of my ordeal is behind me and that the road to recovery has been patched, paved, and plowed. Forgive the mixed metaphor, but there is nothing but smooth sailing in front of me.

Yo-Yo.

You know what one is, right? You wind the string and marvel as the spool goes down and magically climbs back up and into your hand again. If it's something to play with and enjoy, it can be a fun toy.

If you use the term to describe one's health, it takes on a whole different meaning.

On Christmas night, as I climbed under the covers, there was little on my mind except visions of sugar plums dancing in my head. I had no way of knowing it at the time, but I was about to become a human Yo-Yo. Of course, the first challenge was the actual cancer and surgery, (the Yo-Yo goes down) followed by a short reprieve (the Yo-Yo climbs back up) before the blood clots formed. (the Yo-Yo goes down) But I was coming back from the clots. After all, wasn't I able to enjoy Christmas and go for several short walks? (the Yo-Yo climbs back up)

I mentioned it was energizing to socialize with people on Christmas. It helped me to forget my troubles for a few moments. It made me feel normal, and normal made me feel wonderful. Several days after Christmas, a dear friend offered to drop off some books along with another walker and a cane. I was more interested in having some company than I was in the books, so I eagerly accepted her offer. I pictured us having coffee and munching on Christmas cookies. The morning she was to visit, the last Sunday of the year, I woke with a high fever. So much for coffee and cookies as she did make it over but there was no interaction between us. I stayed in the bedroom, buried under a mountain of blankets while she and Marilyn chatted in the living room.

What started as a fever blossomed into a urinary tract infection (UTI). I don't recall ever having a UTI before, but as I was to find out, they are quite impacting as it knocked me on my keister for the next two weeks. (And ...the Yo-Yo goes down).

I was told I could expect to lose weight following my surgery, and I did. Knowing this, I ate with impunity in the days and weeks leading up to the procedure. If it wasn't moving, I jammed it down my gullet. I went into the surgery weighing 216 pounds, by far the heaviest I've ever been in my life. Following my surgery, until New Year's Day, I watched as my weight dropped; slowly at first. Food meant little to me; steak and lobster wouldn't have whetted my appetite. In the first week following surgery, I lost a couple of pounds. No one is going to get too knotted up over losing two or three pounds.

One month later, during the week prior to Christmas, I went for a second follow up visit. My weight at that time was 193lbs. I had now lost 23lbs in the 6 weeks since my surgery date. OK, so now this does have my attention, but I was warned that there would be weight loss so this is not unexpected. I am curious to know what the peak loss will be. I remember having lost somewhere around 35-40lbs in 2007 during my first go around with cancer. My hope is that my weight loss won't get as bad as that.

I do wish food tasted better to me. There is an unpalatable metallic taste in my mouth which makes food and drink taste pretty bad. I eat because I know I have to and not because I'm hungry or have a craving for anything. If food tasted better, I'm sure I'd be inclined to eat more. Marilyn has the unenviable task of getting me to eat. She would love nothing more than to make me a seven course dinner, including all of my favorites. She offers often; I thank her but politely decline. I drink Boost and eat peanut butter and jelly sandwiches. I know I should be taking in 1800-2000 calories a day, but I come nowhere near to that mark.

As mentioned, I was blindsided with a urinary tract infection before New Year's, which laid me out for two weeks. My appetite, which was already bad, disappeared almost entirely while I staved off this infection.

The third week of January, I have another follow up visit. It has been about a month since I last made the trek to the hospital for a visit. Ten weeks, more or less, have passed since my surgery. I weigh in during this consultation at 183lbs. I have now lost 33lbs since my surgery. It's not a good weight loss. No one is saying, *"Hey, you look good. Have you lost weight? You have really slimmed down nicely."*

I look like shit. I know this. My legs look like toothpicks. My arms are scrawny, and the muscle I did have has gone missing. That, Dear Reader, gives you a visual of how I am doing physically at this point, but there is an emotional battle going on at the same time. I'm convinced that the physical and the emotional are playing against one another. The relationship between the two is symbiotic. As my strength and stamina diminish, it gets more difficult to keep on top of my emotions. I find myself weeping, sometimes uncontrollably, multiple times a day. Often this happens for no reason at all.

I discuss this with God. I tell Him that if He wants to call me home, I will go with Him gladly. I don't pray that He'll take me; I just want Him to know that the topic is open to discussion.

On one January day, the reason for my sadness was all too apparent. I mentioned earlier in the book that we were having a really bad cancer year as several friends had been diagnosed with, and were being treated for cancer.

A dear friend, who was my age, retired in the spring. He lived in the neighborhood, and he accompanied me on several walks in the woods with Abbey. I have fond memories of these walks as we talked about anything and everything. He was a very intelligent man, and the conversations were typically stimulating. We were together at a friend's home for a brunch in September, and I noticed my friend had lost weight. His wife, too, looked like she had also lost weight. She called the house a day or two after the brunch, and I asked her what she and her husband were doing to drop weight. I assumed she would say dieting, but her answer surprised me and concerned me. As it turned out, she was dieting which accounted for her weight loss, but she went on to say that her husband was at the hospital at that very moment where they were trying to figure out why he was losing weight. He was given a battery of scans, and labs, and tests, and MRIs. The result of all these tests was not only cancer but multiple cancers. We all tried to be positive about these results and his prognosis, but it didn't sound good from the very beginning.

Marilyn and I bonded fiercely with our friend and his wife. Why wouldn't we? Cancer is horrible and nasty and ugly but it will also draw people together. For the next several months, we spoke often. We compared notes on how everyone was doing. We shared feelings and thoughts and prayers with one another. We leaned on one another. We freely shared both our tears and our fears. Every conversation ended with, 'Let us know if you need anything. If there is anything we can do for you; just ask'.

The offers were sincere, but at the end of the day, we couldn't give our friends what they needed the most.

Then one Saturday morning in mid-January our doorbell rang. Three friends were there to tell us that our friend had passed away. They knew how close we had grown with this poor man and his wife, and they wanted to make sure the news was delivered in a sensitive and personal way. With news like this, no matter how we were told, it was going to be devastating. It all seemed so unfair, but who ever said cancer played fairly? How does a healthy man go from losing weight in September to leaving this world behind in January?

Given my fragile emotional state, I was crushed by the news. I wept for days and then wept some more. My tears were for the loss of a friend, but they were also for the guilt that goes along with surviving when someone else hasn't. I was angry. I was convinced that somehow my friend and I would both survive our cancers. Come springtime, we would once again walk the forest trails together with Abbey in tow. Cancer is a thief and it had stolen that from both of us.

So, as mentioned earlier, I visit the hospital during the third week of January for a follow up. I have prepared a list of questions and concerns to discuss with the doctor. Hopefully, there is a lesson there for anyone going to visit a doctor for any reason. Give thought to what you want to ask and discuss with your doctor and write it out so you don't forget anything. Otherwise, I can almost guarantee that on the way home from the visit you will remember something you forgot to ask about. Trust me; I speak from experience on that point.

One of the items for discussion on my list is hip pain. I'm having trouble straightening my left leg and it is getting more and more difficult to walk. It is almost impossible to find a comfortable position; whether sitting, standing, or lying down. I am assured that this is a common side effect, and I can expect to feel better soon.

But I don't feel better soon. In fact, I feel worse, and then, even worse still. Several days after my visit, I reach out to my nurse to tell her the pain has gone from bad to unbearable. I can barely stand. I walk hunched over at the waist in an effort to take some pressure off the hip. Marilyn borrows a shower bench so that I can sit while I bathe. I tell my nurse about the doctor's claim that the hip pain was considered normal, but this can't possibly be considered normal.

As it turns out, really, as luck would have it, I am scheduled for a post-cancer CT scan several days later. This scan is to determine if my cancer is still in check. The scan will also include the hip area, which may offer some insight into what is causing the pain.

My son took me for my scan, and when I returned home, I immediately climbed into bed. I wasn't tired. I hoped that if I could fall asleep, it might help take my mind off the pain. Several hours later, my wife wakes me from my blessed slumber. It turns out that there is nothing normal about the pain I have been experiencing as the scan shows what is labelled as a pelvic abscess. This is new to me. I had heard of a tooth abscess before but did not realize that they could occur in other parts of the body. I am told that I will need to go to the hospital immediately. I will be admitted. While waiting in the admission area, I Google (Yep, good old Dr. Google) *pelvic abscess*. The first comment I stumble across is, '*A pelvic abscess is a life-threatening collection of infected fluid*'.

Life threatening?!?

Well, I sure don't like the sound of that.

In case you are wondering, Dear Reader, the Yo-Yo is once again on the way down. I will spend the next six days in the hospital. The first thing they do is install a drain into the abscessed area which will allow this infected fluid to exit the body. There is a tube, similar to aquarium hosing for those who ever owned fish, which protrudes from my side. The tube is connected to a bulb which will collect the fluid. It seems to be working as the bulb collects quite a bit of fluid and needs to be emptied often. The fluid is, in a word, gross. I'll leave it at that for my more sensitive readers.

I am lying in my hospital bed and next to my bed is an I-V pole. The purpose of this pole is to hold intravenous concoctions that are being fed into my body. I'm shocked by the number of bags that are hanging off this pole. Each bag has a tube extending from it that is connected to one of the multiple ports that have been installed into my arms and my hands. It would be difficult to find space to fit another bag onto this I-V pole. Everyone seems to be taking this whole abscess thing very seriously as my body is being bombarded by what I believe to be every antibiotic known to man.

Six days later, I am released from the hospital, even though my living room will become an extension of my hospital room. The tube is still draining the infected fluid into the collection bulb. Marilyn and I will be managing this going forward. We will be responsible for emptying the bulb and recording the amount of fluid that has drained. The fluid is now mostly clear so this task isn't too disgusting. I still have quite a bit of hip pain, and so I ask about this. It seems to me that once most of the fluid has been removed, the pain would disappear. Unfortunately, it isn't that simple, as there is more healing that needs to happen in the pelvis. I focus on the fact that the pain is reduced. I am getting better and treat this as a victory. I focus on the same goal I have had since the beginning; *concentrate on feeling better today than you did yesterday.*

Because I had so many I-V tubes connected to me, they installed what is called a PICC (Peripherally Inserted Central-line Catheter) line into my arm. This port will take the intravenous medicine and deposit it into a more major vein closer to the heart. I still have the PICC line when I'm released from the hospital, and as it turns out, I'm not done using it yet. Marilyn and I are responsible for administering an intravenous antibiotic daily via the PICC line. I'm somewhat comfortable with this device as I had a PICC line all summer, which was how my chemo was delivered. I would watch the nurses flush the port and then hook up my big bag of chemo-fun. Marilyn, on the other hand, is totally freaked out the first time she has to help with this. I walk her through it and within a day or two she reaches her comfort level in performing this task. I nickname her *Nurse Marilyn*, but in truth, I don't think Marilyn has the nurse gene in her DNA.

Ten days later, we have administered the last dose of in-home I-V antibiotic. More good news, the bulb has collected negligible amounts of abscess fluid over the past several days. The best news of all is that my hip pain is close to being 100% gone. I go for another CT scan. This scan isn't meant to look for cancer. The purpose is to see if the abscess has healed. The day after the scan, I consult with an infectious disease doctor, who tells me I am at the point where the drain and the PICC line can be removed. I make an appointment to visit my nurse in clinic. She will be responsible for removing the drain and the PICC line. I wish I could tell you, Dear Reader, that I skipped into the clinic that day but the truth is I was still so unsteady on my feet that

I didn't trust myself to even use a walker. Instead, my friend, who had brought me to my appointment, had to use a wheelchair to get me to the nurse's office.

Having these devices protruding from your body is always going to feel alien. Having them removed makes me feel reborn. The Yo-Yo is on the way up, and I believe in my heart that the worst is behind me.

Chapter Twenty-Two: Hospital Stays

Before we move on, I wanted to talk about hospital stays. I have never spent time in a hospital where I haven't come home without a story. These stories aren't profound or poignant; they are typically weird or funny or, in one case, kind of scary. I only had the extravagance of a single bed room once in all my stays. Having a room all to your lonesome is fantastic, but it doesn't lend itself to a good story. If you want to look into the disturbing psyche of a complete stranger in a short period of time, share a hospital room with them. This is not to imply that all of my roommates were head-cases; just most of them.

Years ago, during my first hospital stay, I not only shared a room with someone, we were also expected to share a television. As I wasn't sure what the proper etiquette was, I let him have control of the television most of the time. This seemed like a good idea as this was to be the first of many hospital patients that I shared a room with that talked to themselves. I'm not a psychoanalyst, but in my opinion, nothing screams crazy like a person talking to himself. One evening there was a show that I did want to watch. When I tuned to it, he immediately asked, "What is this crap? I don't want to watch this crap." I successfully ignored him, but this did confirm my already strong suspicion that my bunkmate was coo-coo. I believe his family knew this as they kept apologizing for him. I assured them that everything was fine even though I kept hoping my bunky would be released soon.

He was.

But this clued me into another bizarre thing that happens during a hospital stay. It seems like everyone is intent on making sure your sleep is continually interrupted. When this guy was released, they sent the custodian in at one-in-the-morning to clean the room in preparation for the next patient. Did he try to make as little noise as possible seeing as how it was the middle of the night and there was a sick patient in the room? No, he did not. In fact, it sounded like a marching band was playing on the other side of that thin curtain. Every light in the place was turned on, including some spotlights that were brought in for the occasion.

171

As you might expect, it's not always easy to sleep in a hospital. You're in a strange bed. It's difficult to get comfortable. There's a lot of activity going on around you. All that being said, I'm convinced that there is a device at the nurse's station that alerts them to when a patient has finally drifted off to sleep. When this alarm goes off, that's their cue to spring into action. The lights go on as their oversized computer cart bangs into everything in the room multiple times.

"Hello, Mr. Drnaso. I'm here to check your blood pressure."

My blood pressure? My guess is that it is probably going to be higher than it was a moment ago when I was sound asleep, I think to myself. Besides, haven't they already checked my blood pressure every half-hour since I was admitted, or is that just my imagination? I fully expect them to tell me that they will be back to double check my blood pressure just as soon as they are convinced that I have fallen back to sleep.

My intention in this chapter is not to rank out nurses. I have way too much respect for them to do that. I've been quoted often as saying I'd rather have a good nurse than many of the doctors I've dealt with in my life. Nurses are in the trenches every day with the patients. They listen better. Many have a terrific sense of humor; well, the ones who laugh at my jokes do anyway. They get to know us as people and not just as patients. They often form strong bonds with their patients in the short time that we have together. God bless you for being on the frontline every day ...and all through the night, too.

One of my room mates was truly and certifiably insane. He was saying some odd things when they brought him in and it just got weirder from there. When it was finally just the two of us in the room, he called out to me, "Hey, who's on the other side of this curtain?"

"My name is Chris," I told him.

"Chris? Oh yeah, my wife knows all about you, Chris," he told me.

What the hell did that mean?

It took me a while to realize he wasn't always talking to me when he said something, which was odd as we were the only two people in the room.

172

When he would say something, I decided it was in my best interest to not reply. At one point he started calling me Joe.

"Hey Joe," he called to me, "is there a security guard on your side of the curtain?"

When I told him, no, he told me we were going to have to get out of the room from my side. I didn't really want to respond, but I felt that I should remind him that we were on the seventh floor.

I listened as he carried on a conversation with someone only he could see. That was the point where I started worrying about my own safety. I wasn't sure if he was capable of getting out of the bed, but if he was, I worried that he might come by me. He could have an ax to grind with me. After all, in his delusional state, he believed his wife knew all about me.

Thank God the nurses figured out that something wasn't right. It was probably about the third or fourth time he screamed, "NURSE!" at the top of his lungs. They asked him if he was hallucinating. He told them, no, which I knew was not true. I felt better when they moved him to a room across the hall. Every once in a while I would hear him scream for the nurse. I was OK with that; at least he wasn't in my room anymore.

Another roommate told me he was leaving. It was in the middle of the night. This declaration came with a string of profanities. He sounded angry when he said it. I could hear him making preparations for his breakout. He wasn't in his right mind, so I thought the Christian thing to do was to use my call button to alert the nursing staff to what was going on. When the nurse's aide appeared at my bedside, and asked me what I needed, I told her that my bunkmate was planning his very own *Shawshank Redemption*. She told me I should only use the call button if I needed something, and I shouldn't concern myself with what was happening in the next bed. Message received. As it turns out, my roommate was all talk as he never did make a break for it.

One of my hospital mates was suffering from severe gastrointestinal issues. The man was in tremendous pain and had been wheeled out of the room several times for various tests. In addition, he was seriously overweight. This hospital allowed patients to call down and order their own food. He, too, like most of my other roommates would talk to himself. When he returned from a test, I would hear him say, "Maybe I should order a little something to eat. I think I'll feel better if I eat something." Following that, I would listen as he ordered two of everything on the menu. Shortly after that his gut would start barking at him and then the moaning would start. This ritual repeated itself several times over the next couple of days. I actually liked this guy. He had a huge family, quite literally as they were all on the hefty side. They were all loud, too, and reminded me of a cast from a sitcom.

Hospital stays, even under the best of circumstances, are never going to be all that pleasant, but there seems to be a movement to improve the quality of one's visit. Newer hospitals oftentimes have single patient rooms, which is a luxury. During a recent stay, my room was incredible. It was huge and had a sofa and a lazy boy for the comfort of my visitors. Meal times were at the discretion of the patient. I had the freedom to call and place a food order at any time, similar to ordering room service in a hotel. There was a lot to choose from, and the food was really pretty good. If I wasn't sick, my stay would have been even better. I guess you can afford to offer these amenities when you charge $30.00 for an aspirin. Just sayin'.

At the end of my six-day hospital stay for my pelvic abscess, our younger son, Nick, offered to pick me up and get me home. As you can imagine, after six-days I was anxious to see the hospital in my rear view mirror. Being told you are going home, and actually being released from the hospital, are two different things. There seems to be a lot of delays built into the process of leaving a hospital. This time the process seemed to go pretty smoothly. Perhaps the hospital was as anxious to see me go as I was to leave. When Nick arrived, I asked if he would fetch my clothes from the closet I shared with my roommate. I wanted to be packed and dressed and ready to scoot when I got the final OK to leave. Nick came back with my coat and my shoes. Alright, that was a good start. Now all I needed were pants, shirt, sweatshirt, hat and gloves to complete the ensemble, and that's where the problem started. He informed me that none of those items were in the closet; the cupboard was bare.

174

"Are you sure?" I asked stupidly.

He was.

As I sat on the edge of the bed in my underwear, Nick went to the nurse's station. They too looked in the closet, but had no better luck than Nick did in finding my clothes. There are not a lot of places to look for things in a hospital room, so the search didn't take long.

It's winter in Chicago, so the idea of going home in my underwear is probably not going to work. The nurses feel bad that my clothes have gone missing, so when I ask if they might be able to provide me with a pair of surgical scrubs, they quickly secure a set. Nick helps me get into the pants, but laughs as I go to pull the shirt over my head. It appears to be an extra small. It might fit a third grader but there is no way I'm going to struggle into this shirt. At this point, I don't care. I have pants and that's really the most important thing. I'm bare-chested under my winter coat as Nick exits the hospital parking lot.

I'm cold as I have no shirt on under my coat. I'm used to this as hospitals like to set the thermostat on the lowest setting. I'm not sure why hospitals are typically freezing; they just are.

I'm not worried about any of this. All I'm focused on is that I'm on my way home and that feels pretty damn good.

I believe it is safe to say that when you are admitted to a hospital, your first priority is to be released from the hospital as quickly as possible. So, if I'm right, and you are on a mission to get out of the hospital, you may want to read, study, and memorize 'Chris' Tips on How to Get Released':

First, when they ask you if you are in pain, say no. If they offer you anything, just ask for a couple of Tylenol. Keep in mind, when they remove your bladder, they will gut you like a fish. Was I in pain? Hell, yes, I was in pain, but I was on a mission to get out as soon as possible. The first two days following surgery they gave me Oxycodone and Morphine, both of which knocked me on my buttocks. On day three, once I had regained some semblance of coherence, I asked for nothing more than Tylenol for pain management. I had another reason for just wanting the Tylenol and that was because the powerful opiates they gave on those first two days scared me. I worried that I would leave the hospital as an addict and start robbing convenience stores to feed my cravings. Yes, Tylenol was certainly the prudent choice. Perhaps Marilyn could be a Bonnie to my Clyde.

Second, the nurses will ask you if you want to take a walk. Trust me, the last thing in the world that you want to do is take a walk. You want to ask them if they are out of their minds for even suggesting such a ridiculous thing. Don't question them. Instead, tell them that there is nothing you would like more than to take a walk. A walk sounds like an enchanting idea and you are glad that they suggested it. Don't worry about the angry jagged incision that crosses your entire belly. Even though you are terrified that the stitches will fail and your insides will spill out, you just suck it up and go for a walk.

Third, POOP! Everyone in the hospital from the doctors and the nurses all the way down to the guy that delivers your food tray appear to have a poop fixation. They seem to think there is nothing odd about starting a conversation with the question, "So, have you had a bowel movement today?" This is a hot topic of conversation as they will continue to enquire about the status of that particular bodily function.

You may be able to mask your pain level by just asking for Tylenol, and you may be able to paste a smile on your face when they take you for a walk, but you can't fake this. I guess if I was thinking ahead I could have stopped at a novelty shop and bought some fake doo-doo but that probably wouldn't have been such a great idea. Plus, I don't think it would have fooled anyone.

Flatulence, to my medical team, was almost as exciting as poop as they were thrilled when I told them I was passing gas. If they got that amped up about a fart, I can't imagine what they would do if they won the lottery.

These tips are worth more than the price of the book, but I have to warn you; use them cautiously. There are times that the best place for you to be is in the hospital no matter how much you'd like to go home. For instance, let's say you are bleeding profusely from an open wound; now that may be a good reason to stay hospitalized.

Chapter Twenty-Three: Are we there yet?

I have been writing with the intention of catching you up to where I am at today. I mentioned that this wasn't the ending I wanted to write for my book. Reading back over these last few chapters, it is all just a litany of one setback followed by some brief respite before I was waylaid by my next setback. Cancer keeps throwing left hooks at me, and I keep leaning into them. In truth, it hasn't made for a fun write for me or a very interesting read for you.

For those asking, "'Are we there yet?'", I'm happy to announce that I think we are getting close, but before we cross the finish line, I have one more descent of the Yo-Yo to tell you about. This one is unpleasant to think about or to talk about, but I've been open and honest with you up to this point, and I don't want to deviate from that at this late stage of the book.

Have you ever heard of something called C-Diff?

Neither had I.

The full name is Clostridium Difficile, and according to Doctor Google, it is a bacterium that can cause symptoms ranging from diarrhea to life-threatening inflammation of the colon. I'm getting tired of Dr. Google telling me that I have yet one more potentially life threatening event to deal with.

Let's review:
- Bladder cancer ...potentially life threatening
- Blood clots ...potentially life threatening
- Pelvic abscess ...potentially life threatening
- C-Diff ...potentially life threatening
- Getting out of bed in the morning ...potentially life threatening

Let me be the first to say that these 'potentially life threatening' caveats are getting to be total bullshit.

My C-Diff escalated slowly, so one evening when I pooped, I didn't think much about it. Truthfully, when you're 67 years old, and have a bowel movement, it is often considered a cause for celebration. Ooops, I pooped again. Still no cause for alarm, and then, son-of-a-gun, I pooped again…and again…and again.

By the next morning, this had blossomed into rampant diarrhea.

All right, by now you have figured out why I would have preferred to simply leave this part out of the book. I promise that we will get through this as quickly as possible.

Fast forward; it is twenty-two days later, followed by yet one more course of antibiotics, before my diarrhea had finally started to slowly subside. OK, I'm never shy about making sophomoric jokes so here goes, *twenty-two days of diarrhea can really take a lot out of a person.* Yes, I understand, that was bad even by my low standards.

As it turns out, C-Diff isn't inclined to let people off the hook even after twenty-two days of pooping your brains out. One friend told me his son swore he was still feeling the effects many months later. Another friend told me his brother suffered from it for over a year. After going through multiple courses of antibiotics, he finally was given something called a fecal transplant, and no, I am not making that up, and yes, that is every bit as disgusting as it sounds. It may have been disgusting for him, but it did work.

It has been close to one-month since I finished my antibiotics and my system is nowhere close to being right yet. As with everything, my goal with C-Diff is to try and feel better today than I did yesterday. That would be easier if I didn't panic every time I was more than ten-feet away from the bathroom.

Do you want to hear something weird?

Of course you do.

When I read the warning label on the antibiotic that I was prescribed for C-Diff, it stated, 'May Cause Diarrhea'. I should probably make a comment about that, but I think it stands on its own just fine. It might help you to picture me with a thought bubble over my head with the letters WTF in it.

Why would I tell you about this? Because I have grown attached to you, Dear Reader, and have tried to educate wherever I can throughout this book, so PLEASE keep the following in mind with the hope you might avoid C-

Diff. Wash hands thoroughly after using the bathroom. If you have diarrhea, either use a separate bathroom or clean the bathroom before anyone else uses it. Here's a scary thought, there is an excellent possibility that the C-Diff bacteria is in your home right now at this very moment. It's pretty much everywhere. You should be using this time to clean and sanitize your home, but instead, you're sitting there reading this stupid book. OK, don't panic just yet. If you are a relatively healthy person, you can come into contact with C-Diff bacteria and suffer no ill effects.

So why, after a lifetime of being in the same room as C-Diff, was I suddenly affected by this bacteria? As it turns out, if you have recently been prescribed antibiotics, your chances of being impacted by C-Diff increases. I mentioned that I was bombarded with antibiotics when fighting off my pelvic abscess infection. This is most likely what caused my C-Diff issues. When I discussed this with a friend, he told me that he had once gone through two weeks of diarrhea. This occurred after an oral surgery in which he was given antibiotics. I'm not a doctor, but the more he told me about his symptoms, the more it sounded like C-Diff to me.

It was at the end of this ordeal, and calling C-Diff an ordeal is not overstating it by the way, that my weight loss reached its peak. I now weigh 44lbs less than I did on the morning that I went into surgery five months earlier. I did the math; never trust my math by the way, but I weigh 20% less now than I did five months ago. Earlier in the book I talked about how nothing, even cancer, is all bad, and I gave the example of the cancer diet as being a great way to lose weight. I rest my case.

This wasn't the last descent of the Yo-Yo, but it is the last that I'll share with you as I am feeling a bit worn out. I've run the marathon; I've gone my fifteen rounds, and I'm just really tired at this point. I guess I could delay finishing this book in case there are more ascents and descents of the infernal Yo-Yo, but I don't think I want to do that.

I've put you through enough, and it's time to move on. It's time we cross the finish line together whether my fight with cancer is finished or not.

I realize that it is five months after my surgery, and I still have a ways to go before I'll feel completely recovered. This leads me to ask, "How good can I expect to feel?"

What will the new normal be?

I'm not sure, even though I do know a few things. The obvious one is the bag. I'm having a hard time wrapping my head around the fact that a bag hanging off my side to collect urine is now part of the new normal. Before I started chemo this past summer, I was sent to an audiologist to have my hearing tested and assessed because one of the chemo cocktails I was being given would negatively impact my hearing. My hearing, which was already bad, has gotten worse. This is now part of the new normal. During treatment, I was asked often if I was feeling any numbness in my hands and feet. All summer, as I went through chemo, I could honestly say that, no, I did not feel any numbness. Many, many months later, I mentioned to my oncologist that I was having chronic numbness in my feet. I was told that another chemo drug I was given causes nerve damage in these extremities. What can be done about it? Nothing, the damage to my feet, like the damage to my hearing, is permanent. This, too, is now part of the new normal.

Cancer leaves its patients with 'souvenirs'. These souvenirs are like tattoos in their permanence. Will there be more? I sure hope not but time alone will answer that question.

I talked a lot about normal during this chronicle and up to this point it has been centered on how cancer and cancer treatment impacts normal. Now in the spring of 2020 the entire world is seeking some sense of normalcy.

Before I put this book to bed, I think it's important to talk about the COVID19 Corona virus. This virus has changed each of our lives; perhaps forever. Terms, never heard before, like 'social distancing' and 'sheltering in place' are now part of the daily lexicon.

When I was a young man, in the late sixties and early seventies, the nightly news would begin by giving the daily death tolls from Viet Nam. It was a sad and sick ritual as the number of captured and wounded and killed would be broadcast to the country and the world. Now, decades later, the nightly news is once again tasked with updating the world on the carnage done by the Corona virus.

How many have been newly diagnosed?

How many have died?

We are continually warned to stay at home and to wash our hands thoroughly and often. Traditional every day errands now need to be well planned and thought out. Going to the grocery store is potentially life threatening. Marilyn and I have taken to shopping for groceries online and having them delivered. When they arrive, we open the garage door where a table has been set up. The groceries are placed on the table, and when the delivery man leaves, Marilyn or I go into the garage with gloves and a facemask and wipe everything down with antiseptic wipes. There is zero interaction between us and the delivery man. This is now normal.

The thought of going to a hospital for any reason is downright terrifying. If you are admitted to a hospital, you will not be able to have visitors. There are numerous heartbreaking stories of a loved one going to the hospital, where they pass away. Families aren't given the chance to say good bye or sit and hold their hand during their final hours. There is no goodbye kiss or an opportunity to whisper in their ear that you love them. Burial services can only be attended by ten people, all of whom are wearing masks and surgical gloves and keeping the requisite distance of six-feet between them. Embraces, hugs, and even handshakes are strictly verboten. This is now normal.

Many have taken to wearing surgical masks and gloves, even when taking a stroll outside. We are told to maintain a minimum distance of six-feet from everyone. The grocery stores have tape on the floor at the deli counter and at the checkout lanes to help people keep a safe distance from one another. This is now normal.

Parks are closed.

Beaches are closed.

Restaurants are closed.

Dentist offices are closed.

Elective surgeries have been postponed.

People are stranded on cruise ships with no ports open to them.

Airplanes, the few that are flying, are mostly empty.

There will be no opening day for baseball this year.

March Madness has been cancelled.

Schools are closed. E-Learning is the norm.

Millions have lost their jobs.

Non-essential businesses have been forced to close their doors.

Many manufacturing businesses have abandoned their core business and begun making plastic face shields and masks with the dual purpose of keeping their employees working and also to provide this much needed personal protective equipment to those at risk. Auto manufacturers have retooled and are now producing ventilators.

All of this is part of the new normal.

Marilyn and I are blessed as we are both retired and have the ability to follow the rules and guidelines set up by organizations like the World Health Organization (WHO) and the Center for Disease Control (CDC). Not everyone is as fortunate as we are. Every day thousands of doctors, nurses, police and firemen, along with mail carriers, store clerks and delivery drivers are risking their lives to provide the rest of the world with healthcare and protection and groceries.

People on the wrong side of sixty, with pre-existing medical issues, are considered high risk. I know that includes me. Fear and hyper-paranoia make following the guidelines essential for us. I have no problem spending everyday hidden away in my home as the thought of leaving my home scares me. Corona scares me.

Nursing homes and care facilities are a hot bed for the COVID19 virus as they house so many high risk residents. The care workers in these facilities are also at a greater risk and each day there are more reports of one of these workers contracting the virus or worse yet, succumbing to it.

The questions of when this will end, and how this will end, go unanswered. The idea of walking into a crowded restaurant or tavern is unthinkable. It's hard to picture a day when we will be able to attend a sporting event. As of this date, over 4 million people in the world (over 25% from the US) have been affected. Globally, 281,000 have died from the disease. Eighty thousand in the US have fallen victim to the infection. These numbers are startling when looked at from the point of view that a scant five months ago, on New Year's Day, most of the world had never heard of COVID19.

It is a devious virus. It can attach itself to a person while not making the person sick. This asymptomatic carrier can then infect countless other people. There is no vaccine or antibiotic that will kill the virus. There is no cure. The younger and stronger you are, the better your chances will be to beat this disease, but there are no guarantees for anyone.

Thank you for bearing with me as I included this short section on COVID19. I didn't include this information for those reading this book in 2020 as everyone on the planet is well aware of this virus and the devastation that it has visited upon the world. This segment is for future generations, so that they may know and understand what life is like for us today.

But let us continue lest we lose our way along the path we have travelled together. This chapter title asked the question, "Are we there yet?" I think we are, or at least we are getting really close.

Thank you for staying with me while I chronicled my cancer journeys. At the risk of repeating myself once again, let me say this is a book I never thought I'd write, but as the saying goes, here we are. As I told you my story, I may not have always been brave or courageous on this journey, but I have tried my best to be open and honest.

I am not the brightest guy in the world, but I am smart enough to know that I have been blessed. Cancer takes people out of this world every day, and even though cancer has had a field day with me for the past fourteen years; I am still standing. Knowing this, I'd be a fool to not acknowledge the blessings that have been bestowed upon me.

I feel like I need to say something inspirational or profound to wrap things up but the words aren't coming to me. Maybe the following will suffice.

I can tell you that Cancer Sucks. I'm sure you've heard that expression before, and I believe there is truth in it.

There are days when Cancer Sucks the hope out of a person.

There are days when Cancer Sucks the strength out of a person.

There are days when Cancer Sucks the laughter out of a person.

There are days when Cancer Sucks the will to live out of a person.

There are days when Cancer Sucks the spirit out of a person.

There are days when Cancer Sucks the fight out of a person.

And there are days, really bad days, when Cancer Sucks someone we love right out of our lives. They're there one moment, and then they are gone. It's easy to hate cancer, but it is especially easy to curse cancer on those days. Sadly, I believe most people who read this book have had a really bad cancer day at one point in their life; a day when someone you love is no longer with you.

So what about your much beleaguered author?

What will become of this sad pathetic scribe?

I guess I'll go on fighting the good fight as well as I can for as long as I can. There are days when that task seems daunting; days that I really don't want to carry on the battle, but I will. There's no way that I'm going to let that bully cancer off the hook that easily. As many times as he comes for me, I'll be ready for him. I will brace myself; I will grit my teeth and carry on the fight until there is no more fight in me. And in the end, if cancer finally does take me down, I promise you that this most despicable of all enemies will know that he's been in a fight.

A Brief Afterword

Hello again! There are always delays when publishing a book and this time has been no different. As several weeks have gone by, I thought I'd give you a quick update.

I went for my CT scan. This is the test that shows if cancer has come a callin' again, and I'm happy to tell you that the news is good. No new cancer. My oncologist described the results as 'unremarkable', and I wish I could tell you this was the first time in my life that I was described as unremarkable, but alas. Of course that was a stressful day. In six-months I'll be sent for another scan.

Thank you all, once again, for taking the cancer journey with me.

The End
C. Drnaso
2020

Chris Drnaso

Acknowledgments

Once again, I am so grateful to the people in my life who are willing to help by reading, proofing, and commenting on my writing.

To my dear wife **Marilyn**, my best friend and tireless caregiver. Your dedication to me means the world to me, so how could I not dedicate this book to you?

For my cousins **Dan and Gloria Yakes**. My computer did not like the five month hiatus I was on. Thank you for breathing new life into an old machine, and of course, thanks for your encouragement and your feedback.

Thank you **Craig Hergenroether,** another dear friend from decades ago. Craig you are not only a great friend and devoted grandfather, you are also a skilled editor and proofreader. As I write this, Craig and I are both anxiously awaiting his test results. I love you, brother.

I may have mentioned in every book I've ever written that I have an awesome sister. **Pat Koche**, I know you love me dearly and that it was difficult at times for you to read about your brother's trials in CANCER BABBLE. Thank you once again for your help with proofing and editing. And this time around, I also have to thank **Richard Koche**, my friend and brother-in-law for reading and commenting on this latest work.

I'm excited to report that **Dave Karpowicz,** my oldest friend in the world, now lives back in my extended neighborhood. Well, in truth, he lives about two and a half hours away in Michigan, but that's still a lot closer than Durango, Colorado. Dave, thanks for standing by me through all my works. I value your input. Lunch in St. Joe's, MI. was one of the highlights of my almost normal autumn.

A special thanks to **Pastor Judy Jones** of the United Church of Christ for reading and commenting on my chapter titled, *'Are you out there, Lord?'* Your input meant a great deal to me. Judy and I are both members of the League of Aspiring Writers. I envy your faith and appreciate your feedback.

187

Thank you to **Dr. Cathy MacLean**, for allowing me to quote your article, *'Sharing a Passion, Sharing Resources'*

Thank you to my dear friend **Kathy McHugh** for being at my side during so many of my dark moments. And of course to our mutual friend **Fred Hosteny** who inspired me on my journey as he traversed his own.

On that same theme, my longtime friend **Jerry Muzika** deserves a shout out for his love and devotion. I called you during some rough times and you always got me laughing about something. That's precious.

Thanks to **Mike Hock** and **Lourdes Aguirre** for your input on a very early copy of *CANCER BABBLE*.

Thanks to **Joe Orlandino**, marketing guru, film producer, and caregiver extraordinaire, for reading and commenting on my book and cover.

Thank you to all the doctors, nurses, technicians, and researchers who wake each day ready to battle cancer.

Thank you to all the cancer patients and caregivers who I have met over the years as I drew strength from each of you. A special thanks to those folks who shared their stories with me. Stories that sadly ended up in Chapter Twelve....you know, the chapter about stupid things people say to cancer patients.

I could have dedicated this book to any one of the following. They are all important people in my life who were taken by cancer. Your fight inspired me; you are not forgotten. **Marko D, Pauline W, Joe F, Hank D, Bill C, Randy F, Linda F, Erin F, Sophie W, Patty B, Dave N, Jenny A,** and **Linda H**. I lost two friends to cancer while writing this book **Bob M** and **Milo L**....I miss you both.

And of course, THANK YOU, **My Dear Lord** for the comfort you gave me in my darkest moments. There are no atheists in cancer-land, but of course, you already knew that.

Made in the USA
Monee, IL
22 February 2021

60941045R00115

Who Has the

Power

of the

Purse?

The Guide to the
Federal Budget Process

Patricia D. Woods PhD

The Woods Institute offers seminars for businesses and organizations that need to understand the legislative operations in the U.S. Congress and the state, local, and national government relations within the federal system. Programs are tailored to the interests of the participants. Speakers and course materials are chosen to meet the client's needs. Members of Congress and their staffs, elected state and local officials, journalists, and government scholars are among the speakers who particpate in the Institute's programs. Clients have included Aerospatiale, Bureau of Land Management, Georgetown University, McDonnell Douglas Corporation, National Association of Counties, National Park Service, Naval Air Systems Command, Naval Test Pilot School, Office of Inspector General (Department of Defense), U.S. Conference of Mayors, U.S. Department of State, U.S. Fish and Wildlife Service, USDA Forest Service, U.S. Information Agency, and the University of Virginia.

ISBN 978-1452854588

Additional copies may be purchased from

The Woods Institute
2231 California St., N.W., #603
Washington, DC 20008
(202) 483-6167;
e-mail: pwoods@woodsinstitute.com
www.woodsinstitute.com

Printed in the United States of America